Irresistible
Communication
Creative Skills for the Health Professional

MARK KING, Ph.D.
School of Health Related Professions
University of Pittsburgh

LARRY NOVIK, M.D.
New York City
Attending Physician on Staff at
    Cabrini Medical Center
    Beth Israel Hospital
    Mount Sinai Hospital
    Stuyvesant Polyclinic

CHARLES CITRENBAUM, Ph.D.
Private Practice
Baltimore, Maryland

W. B. Saunders Company
PHILADELPHIA   LONDON   TORONTO   MEXICO CITY   RIO DE JANEIRO   SYDNEY   TOKYO

W. B. Saunders Company: West Washington Square
                        Philadelphia, PA   19105

                        1 St. Anne's Road
                        Eastbourne, East Sussex BN21 3UN, England

                        1 Goldthorne Avenue
                        Toronto, Ontario M8Z 5T9, Canada

                        Apartado 26370—Cedro 512
                        Mexico 4, D.F., Mexico

                        Rua Coronel Cabrita, 8
                        Sao Cristovao Caixa Postal 21176
                        Rio de Janeiro, Brazil

                        9 Waltham Street
                        Artarmon, N.S.W. 2064, Australia

                        Ichibancho, Central Bldg., 22-1 Ichibancho
                        Chiyoda-Ku, Tokyo 102, Japan

Library of Congress Cataloging in Publication Data

King, Mark.
Irresistible communication.

1. Medical personnel and patient.   2. Communication in
   medicine.   I. Novik, Larry.   II. Citrenbaum,
   Charles.   III. Title

R727.3.K56   1982   610.69'6   82-47769

ISBN 0-7216-5429-0

Photographs by Jim Martin

Irresistible Communication   ISBN   0-7216-5429-0

Last digit is the print number: 9   8   7   6   5   4   3

Dedication

Once upon a time, I came across an immense and beautiful forest. It was laden with many paths and many adventures. I chose a path and soon was joined by a Deer and Parrot. The Deer was soft and sweet, but at the same time very strong. The Parrot was powerful and squawked a lot, but was really quite gentle and sensitive. We came to a beautiful Lake and I stayed and drank the Lake's sweet and refreshing water. Then, with the Deer and the Parrot by my side, I took a new path. Sometimes I felt playful and the Deer said, "Play, if that's what you desire." The Parrot disagreed and urged me to earnestly continue on my way. I soon learned that both were right, and I playfully went on. A wonderful Fern grew in the forest and was always present to provide me nourishment. Suddenly I saw myself on the path. It was my image on a Mirror that was hanging on a tree. I took the Mirror with me, was comforted by it, and learned much about myself from its many reflections. I found a magical Jewel and carried that with me also. Now I look at the Jewel often and am fascinated by its deep beauty and by an Aura and Rainbow that surround it. Although my journey through the forest is not finished, I'm thankful for all that I have found there, especially the Deer, for telling me to play, and the Parrot, for urging me on my way.

CMC

Introduction

Wait a second! I thought I was finished with all those irrelevant courses, like Music Appreciation 101. I don't have time for this, I've got to study important things like anatomy. . . .

Sometimes, in the midst of all our studies, we forget what the finished product is supposed to look like. You are actually all preparing for a career as professional communicators. Perhaps at this moment in time you're concentrating on acquiring a broad base of knowledge. Of course, while this is invaluable, it is only a prerequisite for your career as a professional who must interact with patients in such a way that this knowledge makes an impact on them. Some people think that the health professionals' job consists mainly of knowing the correct thing to do and telling it to their patients. If the patients don't respond, it's the patients' fault. Brilliant practitioners can give all the right advice, but if there is noncompliance, they have not achieved a true experience of success. Instead, there are only reasons such as, "that patient doesn't want to get better," or "he's too forgetful," or "he's a stubborn person!"

In this book, we present an alternative approach to the practice of health care, one that promises to bring a great deal more satisfaction to both the patient and the health professional. It gives you the opportunity to take responsibility in your daily patient encounters in such a way that what you really intend to say at every moment reaches and affects that person. Your job is not done until you have a clear perception that the patient's symptom(s) are better. Thus, coming up with the right answer or diagnosis or latest treatment is no longer the "main event"; communicating it so that it becomes useful for the patient *is*. Your intending to communicate in such a way will probably in itself be accompanied by better results in your particular health field.

There are three major difficulties in writing a text such as the one in hand. The first is that in some way the ideas are so simple that when presented in a book as short as this, the reader may rightfully ask, "How can we possibly expect all the changes that you promise to take place with such little detailed information about these techniques?" On the other hand, the ideas in their subtlety are so complex that even 700 pages of written communication would not be able to begin to scratch the surface. We have chosen to make this an introductory text and present these ideas to you believing that this will be your first exposure to some of them (especially the indirect techniques). We firmly believe that even discussed at this introductory level, the use of these effective communication techniques will bring you dramatic results in terms of working with patients. We also know, however, that to become a masterful communicator, it will take more than reading the text. For those of you who are "turned on" by these ideas, we hope that you will be taking more advanced communication courses and spending time in continuing education programs and workshops with effective professional communicators whom you know of or have heard about. Some of the more subtle things, such as body language, are difficult to teach through the written medium.

Another major problem for us is the constitution of language. We need to speak a common language in order to communicate with words. Yet, for professionals, many of the common metaphorical words that we will be using have already been pre-empted by other theoretical schools of thought. A prime example of this is the use of the terms "unconscious" and "conscious." Psychoanalytic psychology has become so much a part of our time that even those of you without a background in the field of psychology and those of you who have never read Freud or any of his followers still have heard of the concept of the unconscious and probablfy have some pretty firm ideas about what that means, As a matter of fact, our understanding of the unconscious is quite different from that of the Freudian perspective. First of all, it and many other terms and concepts we will be using—including physical entities such as the right and left side of the brain—are metaphors that we are not suggesting exist per se. We have all come to use metaphors every day in understanding our world. If a patient or a friend came to you with a "heavy heart," each of you would be able to immediately understand what he or she was saying and would probably not run for your scale in order to weigh it to measure the pathology. Therefore, since we're not in the business of inventing new words, in this text we will be using some of the terms in slightly different ways than you might be familiar with. We know that you have the ability to keep an open mind and adapt to our usage of language and wanted to just take this opportunity to remind you of the many times that you've done it before, and to thank you for your patience and attention.

The last major difficulty for us has been our inability to remember the original sources of all the many stories, patient examples, and even some of the techniques that we discuss in this book. Over the years we have collectively attended a large and unknown number of workshops, read more books than we probably care to remember, and had a voluminous number of informal discussions with helpful and insightful health professionals. Many of the sources of the material will go unnamed, not because we do not remember the particular individuals, but rather because we cannot connect the particular stories or techniques with them. Certainly, throughout the text we have given much deserved credit to Milton H. Erickson, Richard Bandler, and John Grinder. A very high percentage of this text deals with those three individuals' work in psychotherapy, translated here for the use of health professionals.. Some other outstanding professional communicators who have contributed ideas that are not necessarily referenced because of the above-stated problem are Joseph Barber, Paul Carter, William Cohen (whose article is used to end Chapter 4), and Steve Gilligan. We also want to thank the many people who did reviews for our publisher and made many helpful suggestions that were incorporated in the final draft of this text. We do not even know the names of many of these people.

Oh yes, one more thing. If you *are* willing to take the responsibility for having everything you say to patients become an actual part of them, then reading this book will be an exciting challenge rather than a chore. It will simply represent a natural reaction on your part to want to know as much as you possibly can about making a wonderful difference in people's lives. You will equally want to know the most creative and effective communication techniques that are available.

After all, isn't it about time we abandoned this antiquated concept of "patient noncompliance" and instead simply started *creating* compliant patients.

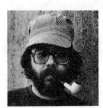

MEK

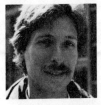

LN

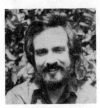

CMC

Contents

IRRESISTIBLE
COMMUNICATION
Creative Skills for the
Health Professional

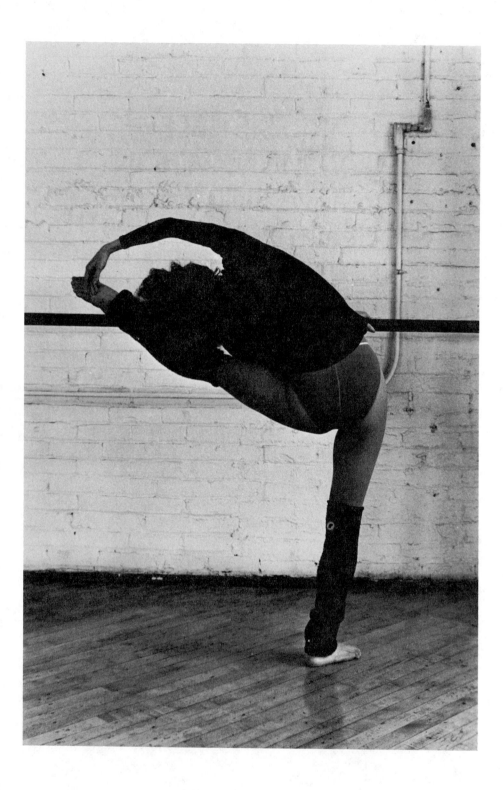

Reality Strategies 1

About a hundred years ago in London the Reverend Edwin Abbott wrote a delightful story called *Flatland: A Romance in Many Dimensions*. *Flatland* is a story of a two-dimensional world that has length and width but no height. Everyone in Flatland moved around freely as shadows would move on the surface of the earth, totally unaware of the dimension of height. The main character in Flatland was a square who one night had a dream that he was transported to Lineland. In Lineland all things were either points or a series of points arranged in a straight line. Everything moved along freely on this one dimension but had no idea of width or height. In Lineland the hero square tried to explain to the characters the missing dimensions. He eventually got so frustrated that he went up to the longest line and said, "Here in Lineland you are the Line of lines, the King of lines; but in my world, in Flatland, you would be nothing. Compared to me you are nothing, and yet I, compared to the nobles in my world, am only a square." Eventually, all the lines got very angry at the square and began to line up their points ready to attack him—when he suddenly awoke from his dream, shaken, but yet happy to realize it was only a dream. Later that day the square was explaining to his grandson, a hexagon, some notations in geometry. (In Flatland, each succeeding generation of males had one more side than its father's until there were so many sides to a figure that it could not be distinguished from a circle, the priestly order. This, of course, was with the exception of the lowly triangles, who will always be triangles.) As the square was explaining to his grandson how to figure out the number of square inches in a square by raising the number of inches on one side to the second power, the grandson asked what it would be like in geometry if something were raised to the third power. The square patiently explained that there was no such thing in geometry as the third power. The grandson, puzzled, kept persisting and eventually the square, angry, sent him to bed, telling him that if he would try to make more sense and talk less nonsense, he would do much better in geometry. Later that night while sitting reading the newspaper, the square kept muttering to himself, "There is no such thing as the third power in geometry." Then all of a sudden he heard a voice saying, "Yes there is!" He looked around and saw a sphere in his living room. The sphere was a visitor from Spaceland, a world that has the three dimensions that we know about here on earth. The sphere tried to explain to the square about Spaceland, and when he was unsuccessful, he created for the square what could be called a transcendental experience; that is, he transported him to Spaceland. The square opened his eyes in Spaceland and looked around and said, "This must be madness or hell." And the sphere said, "It's neither; it's knowledge. Open up your eyes and look around." The square did and, excited about what he found, he started talking to the sphere about the possibility of a world

3

with four dimensions or five dimensions. The sphere said, "There is no such thing," and immediately and angrily threw him back to Flatland. The square went around Flatland preaching the gospel of a world with three dimensions. Not believed, an inquisition eventually confined him to a mental institution where once a year he was visited by the priestly circle asking him how he was getting along, and each time he couldn't help but explain to the circle about Spaceland—at which time the circle shook his head and left for the year. (Abbott, 1952)

THE NATURE OF REALITY

This chapter is about the nature of personal reality. One might ask, Why start out such a practical book, a book about communication for health professionals, with a philosophic discussion about the nature of reality? It is simply because when individuals communicate with one another, what they are trying to communicate is their reality, i.e., their understanding of the world or a particular situation in the world. Therefore, in order to understand anything about effective communication, we must understand something about the nature of reality. Reality is simply what is experienced by an individual. Oftentimes we mistake consensual validation, or what we call truth, with reality. While metaphysics or truth is a very interesting and important issue for philosophers and scientists, for professional communicators it can get in the way if not distinguished from reality. For example, if a patient comes to a doctor experiencing pain, it doesn't do anyone any good to look at the x-ray and see that for that particular disorder, the pain should not be experienced, and therefore to conclude that the pain does not exist or that the pain is only psychologic. The pain is real in that it is actually being experienced by the patient. If the doctor is to effectively communicate with a patient, the doctor has to understand that patient's reality. In our society, we are so concerned with consensual validation that we have relegated some of our most important experiences to the unreal. Dreaming is a good example of this. When you dream, the bear that chases you in the woods is real and the table and chair in the room and the very bed you sleep on are unreal, in that they are not experienced by you. However, we often misunderstand this and think that reality consists only of things that are physical, such as the chair, or of objects that everyone can experience.

There is an old baseball story in which the umpire seems to have a particularly fine knowledge about the nature of reality. When he called a pitch a strike, the manager came out to argue with him. After a few minutes, the umpire ended the discussion by saying the following: "The pitch was neither a ball or strike, it was nothing but a little baseball being thrown by that man standing 60 feet, 6 inches away. The pitch was nothing until I called it, and then it was whatever I called it." In the same way that the pitch was neither a ball nor a strike until the umpire experienced and labeled it, all phenomena are unimportant, and even unreal, until they are experienced by an individual.

All people develop a strategy or group of strategies for understanding the world. We call these reality strategies. Many patients with whom health professionals come in contact have developed strategies that are dysfunctional for them. The major job of health professionals, in terms of communication, is to help alter the reality strategy of their clients. Most clients experience the world as somewhat impoverished, and yet we know that the world is very rich. Therefore, it is not important that we change the world, but only that we help the clients to change their way of viewing the world. Clients often feel "stuck" or "impotent" in their particular life situation, and yet we know that there are a multitude of available options that, if used, would enable them to feel powerful and free.

Some years ago the Denver Zoo had a particularly prized animal in a temporary cage that was too small for it. The animal spent the entire day walking the 60 feet from one end of the cage to the other. One day the cage was lifted so that the animal could live in the large naturalistic environment built around the temporary shelter. When released, the animal kept pacing to where the old bars used to be, stopped, turned around, went the other way, stopped, and turned around again. Like this animal, most of us and many of our patients are in self-imposed cages that limit the richness and possibilities of the world. One major job of health professionals is to help patients understand, and when needed alter, their views of the world in service of a health-related goal.

In the same way that the goal of health professionals is to alter the reality strategies of their clients, the goal of teachers and authors is to alter the reality strategies of their students and readers. Our job in writing this text is to change the view that present and future health professionals have of a particular phenomenon—communication.

ALTERING REALITY STRATEGIES

It has become obvious to us from observing interactions of health professionals and their clients that most clients will believe anything that is congruently transmitted to them by health professionals.* That is why, for example, placebos, witch doctors, and faith healers are so effective in alleviating symptoms for those who believe. This is especially true when the treatment involves a high degree of dependence upon verbal communication. The best example of this is in psychotherapy, where there are a large number of psychotherapists and even a greater number of clients running around believing all kinds of crazy things about themselves. For example, many people today believe they have inside of them somewhere an id, an ego, and a superego. These three parts of the "mind" really do exist for the psychoanalysts and their clients, and

---

*By congruent transmittal, we mean any verbal communication that is supported by appropriate body language and behavior. A common example of noncongruent behavior is telling someone that you are angry with them while at the same time taking a relaxed posture and smiling.

they have been able to use this "reality" (that is, the existence of the id, the ego, and the superego) as part of a strategy to help the patients and themselves understand what is going on and how they can change it. There are many other people walking around today with "parents, adults, or children," with "topdogs and underdogs," and with habits formed from a sequence of rewards or punishments associated with certain stimuli and responses (terms used respectively in transactional analysis, Gestalt therapy, and behavior modification therapy).

Since clients will believe almost any "reasonable" reality presented to them, why not develop a strategy for yourself and your client that says that anyone can change or do almost anything and that they can do it quicker and with more fun and personal reward than they thought possible. This seems to us to be an effective strategy message to convey to clients. One of the reasons why we believe that many helping professionals don't convey such a message is that there is a tendency in all of us to avoid "looking bad." By telling their clients that change will be gradual, slow, and for some people not even possible, they are taking no risk for failure with their client. If change happens more quickly than expected, they look like magicians; if not, they look like the normal, cautious professionals that they sometimes fear themselves to be. This attitude, while being a safe one for health professionals in terms of how they look to the client, is sometimes dysfunctional in terms of therapeutic change.

One of the first important pieces of diagnostic information that you need to discover is the patient's belief in how long it will take for him or her to get better. One way to do this is to tell a few short stories about people who have had similar conditions and about one who got better in a week or so, surprising everyone, another who took 3 or 4 weeks, and another who took 6 months, watching all the while for the patient's nonverbal responses. Usually by little nods and a smile, you will be able to tell what the patient believes it will take in terms of time for him or her to get better. In Chapter 2 we will discuss what to do with this information once you have it.

Remember that for effective communication to occur, it is important that your verbal messages be congruent with the rest of your presence (your body, posture, voice tone, and gestures). Don't slump in your chair and whisper that the client needs to be more assertive. Don't frown seriously as you tell the patient in gait-training apparatus that you think he'll be walking on his own soon. All of us are able to recognize the difference between someone saying, "I love you," either honestly or dishonestly. The honest response is accompanied by a relaxation of the facial muscles, a smile, solid eye contact, and possibly an upturning of the hands. Lying may be accompanied by shifting of the eyes, a monotone delivery, and a "half" smile. Though many of us may not recognize each ingredient in the response, the finished product is usually obvious.

For example, in a case to be discussed in detail in Chapter 7, the authors treated a 20-year-old patient who had severe, persistent allergy, by using a storytelling technique. Even though there was nothing in our experience or the literature indicating success in using this method for this symptom (in fact, we took the client on only because it seemed like an interesting learning experience for us), we told the client we were certain that the symptoms would be gone, probably fairly soon. Even though we knew the probability of looking incompetent was high, any other introductory message would have guaranteed nonproductive results. The best possible results in the health professions occur when the knowledge of modern science is combined with the faith evoked by the shaman.

For the remainder of this chapter, we will be sharing some of our reality strategies about the nature of communication with you. We believe that these are not only highly effective strategies for producing effective communication for health professionals, but they are also good strategies for living an effective life. (As you can see, modesty is not one of our strategies.)

Milton H. Erickson

Before beginning with specific strategies for effective communication, we would like to share more general life strategies that we've learned from three people—Milton Erickson, Richard Bandler, and John Grinder—whose ideas permeate this text. Dr. Milton H. Erickson, who is known as the father of clinical hypnosis, is an unusual man because the difficulties he had to overcome in life were more severe than most of us and, in fact, many of our clients will ever have to face. Twice he was struck by poliomyelitis, once so severely they thought he would never be able to talk again; he had to teach himself to do so, beginning by whistling through gaps in his teeth. Many of the specific strategies to be discussed later in this text will be derived from Erickson's ideas of communication.

Perhaps the most important thing we have gained from spending time with Milton Erickson and reading his work is a particular understanding of life that labels everything that happens unexpectedly, and particularly those things that appear to be initial setbacks of some kind or another, as unprecedented opportunities to learn something new about ourselves and the world. All of us are confronted every day with unexpected events, many of which at first appear to be problematic for us. Think about how important and effective it would be for each of us and, through us, for our clients to learn to look at each of these situations not as a "setback," but rather as an opportunity given to us by whatever forces we believe in to grow, to learn more about ourselves, to learn more about our world, and particularly to learn how we function in unexpected situations. That seems to us to be preferable to the "tape" that most of us run in our minds when something unexpectedly negative or unusual occurs, or when we believe we have an unprecedented opportunity to get anxious, depressed, or angry. If you begin to share Dr. Erickson's "unprecedented opportunity" outlook, you will see how different the world will begin to look.

Bandler and Grinder—"The Modelers"

Richard Bandler and John Grinder, in addition to teaching us some specific communication techniques that will be discussed later, also taught us a very effective strategy for living. These men call themselves "modelers" because they learn by studying people who are effective at what they do. We have learned from them to seek out all people who are great at what they do, not just those in our particular field. For example, one of the authors recently traveled at some inconvenience to another city to watch Andres Segovia give a concert in classical guitar. The author did so, not because he is a great fan of classical music, but because he recognizes Segovia as the best at what he does and therefore knew that by watching carefully he could learn more about things that he himself does—that is, teaching and psychotherapy. We are dedicated to seeking out those people who are very good at what they do, studying their technique, and then applying some of the principles to our own particular areas of interest.

Most creative people in the arts have been considered "bad interviews" by the media. We believe this is because they are content for the most part to sit back and spend a lot of time observing and learning about the world; they do not feel the need to be at the forefront of social events.

OBSERVATION SKILLS

It is challenging to use the written media to help people become better observers. One of the best ways that has worked for us has been to be around

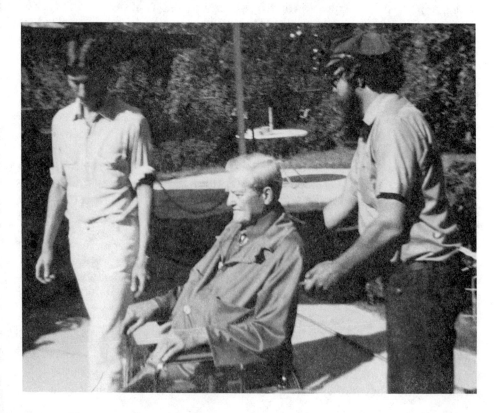

teachers who modeled such behavior. The first hint we can give you is not to make assumptions too quickly about what is going on in a given situation. However clearly you may think you see it, there is almost always an equally viable alternative explanation. For example, since this is a book about communication for health professionals, you might reasonably assume that the picture on page 8 is of two professionals therapeutically communicating with a patient. Can you tell which one of the professionals is the physician? Is the other really a professional or is he a hospital orderly? Actually, the old sick "patient" in the wheelchair is Dr. Erickson, who is doing the effective communicating. Now which one do you think is the patient?

We will now discuss some specific reality strategies that we as health professionals use in understanding and functioning as professional communicators. The first two of these strategies are central to and interact with all of the other techniques discussed later in this book. They are so critical that we are willing to say that if you get nothing out of this book except for these two strategies, you will still have made a great leap forward in becoming an even more effective health professional.

FLEXIBILITY

The first of these strategies is flexibility of approach to each client. Most health professionals learn a particular way of approaching a patient. When that method works, they are to be congratulated because they have done something effective. However, when it doesn't work, most health professionals, in their attempt to communicate with their patients, often try the same thing again, longer and louder. When they finally have tried this approach as long and as loudly as possible and it still doesn't work, they resort to name-calling. They either call their patients names—"resistant" is one of their favorites—or they blame themselves by saying that they are just not powerful enough, that they look too young for the patient to trust them, that they're not well spoken or intelligent looking enough.

Bandler and Grinder have conceptualized a very helpful way to look at this approach. They call it the "Law of Requisite Variety." This principle says that in anything that operates systematically, the element in the system with the most variability will have the most control. Therefore, it is important for communicators to be more varied—that is, more flexible—than their clients. It is clear to us that this is not usually the case with most health professionals. For example, many nurses have learned in school the "professionally proper" way to respond to patients. When they get a behavior management case that does not respond to this "textbook" style of communication, they get stuck and are unable to generate alternative responses.

In psychotherapy, one reason why psychotics have traditionally been seen as difficult to work with is partly because the professional attempting to communicate with them is locked into a certain way of behaving and understanding the world. Yet many types of psychotics are willing to try anything in order to avoid contact, or to get their way, for instance. The client in this case has much more flexibility and freedom in range of expression than the therapist. We also feel that the lack of flexibility by parents is the reason why children have as much power as they do in families. One might ask one's self how little tots, only knee-high and not even able to take care of themselves physically, can have so much power in many families. We believe it is partly because children, at least initially, have more flexibility than their parents. The parents have certain "shoulds" in their heads about what it's like to be a parent, and they often act out these "shoulds" no matter how ineffective their approach. Children, however, are willing to try anything to see if it works. If it works, it is continued; if not, something else is tried until they get their way. In many cases children have more requisite variety or more flexibility than their parents and therefore have much more control than they have a right to have, given their position in the family.

Stated again, the basic principle of flexibility is that you do something that you believe will work and you observe whether or not it works. If it does, you continue to do or say the same thing with whatever modifications are necessary. If it does not, rather than continue in the same approach, you try something different. You do this as often as is necessary for each individual client.

Using this approach presupposes not only the willingness to attempt new ways of doing things but, equally important, the sensory experience of seeing, hearing, and feeling if what you are offering is being accepted. For example, a therapist often doesn't have to wait until the next office visit to see if the patient will really stick to a prescribed diet. By observing the patient closely and listening to the tone and tempo of the patient's actual words, the therapist can make a more educated guess as to the effect of the intended communication. All of us have had the experience of witnessing someone say "yes," and someone else say "YES!" (Say it both ways out loud right now while noticing your accompanying body language.) Not simply the loudness of the utterance, but the quality of tone and tempo, the accompanying (or absent) head nod, the raising of the eyebrows, and the movement of hands, trunk, and shoulders will often give us an intuitive feeling of whether or not the patient is definitely sincere, or congruent, in his or her reply.

Patients are not usually wholeheartedly insincere or deceptive; instead, parts of them are in disagreement with other parts. In our example, one part of the person might really want to lose weight, but another part enjoys eating and all of the positive aspects associated with it. Only if the professional has the full sensory experience necessary to know what type of response is occurring can he or she be confident that the message was communicated effectively or decide that another method must be tried in order to successfully reach the person or the part of the person unresponsive to the message.

An excellent example of requisite variety is illustrated by the following case. Leslie Cameron, a well-known family therapist, was working with a mother, father, and son in front of a large group. No matter how hard she tried, she could not gain control over the family, because the various members continued to argue with each other, making any successful movement impossible. At that point, she could have done one of several things. She might have announced that this was the worst family that she had ever worked with and that she wouldn't waste her time any longer, or she could have started lamenting to herself how she wished she were a more effective therapist. Instead, however, she accurately interpreted the prevailing situation to mean that what she had been doing with those particular people in that particular place and time was not working and that something else had to be tried to secure their attention. At this point, she fell over and faked a seizure. Afterwards, she got back up, restarted the session, and, with the utmost attention and cooperation from the family, was able to conduct a successful therapeutic encounter in the remaining time.

In another example, a nurse came to one of the authors seeking advice about a patient who was constantly angry about hospital issues and policy and who was not very cooperative even in terms of her own treatment. The nurse had tried to reason with the patient and had argued with the patient, without any success in gaining her cooperation. The nurse was asked if she was willing to try something new. She agreed and the next day went storming into the patient's room raving about "the goddamned hospital" and its "_____ policies." Soon the patient and nurse were good friends, and patient cooperation was no longer an issue. (This is also a good example of pacing the client's reality, which will be the subject of Chapter 2.)

If your reality strategy allows you to believe that there is no such thing as a resistant patient who won't get better, and if you can assume that there is no patient whom you can't treat effectively, and if you are flexible and observant enough, then every patient or client who comes to you will have a high probability of successful treatment outcome.

Professionalism Reassessed

Much of our lack of flexibility as professionals comes from an outmoded understanding of the nature of "being a professional." It is not, in our opinion, unprofessional to wear a Superman costume to teach a class if that's what works in getting the class's attention; to walk with a patient to get a beer if that's what is needed to have the patient trust you and begin to take medication regularly; to tell jokes if it will relax a patient in a dentist's chair; or to shout and cuss if that's what motivates the client. It is unprofessional to be stiff and formal with a client who responds better to casualness; to listen politely to the hypochondriac who needs to be told firmly not to call on weekends; or to sit in your office if the best treatment milieu is outside. A good professional attitude occurs when the client's welfare is the guiding motivation for your behavior. A good professional is one who works effectively for the client.

UTILIZATION OF BEHAVIOR

The second major idea or reality strategy that we have used for effective communication is the principle of utilization of behavior. This principle simply states that you take whatever behavior, including verbalizations, that the client gives you and use it in the treatment process. Oftentimes health professionals have set ideas about certain behaviors, especially behaviors we call symptoms. These set ideas say that these are behaviors that we need to eliminate. They are never thought of as being useful in the treatment, even though it is clear by the patient's persistent actions that these are behaviors that are most meaningful to the patient. Perhaps the most striking example of utilization of behavior is given in Jay Haley's book about the work of Milton Erickson, *Uncommon Therapy* (1973). One day, while working in a mental hospital, Erickson was assigned a patient who believed himself to be Jesus Christ and had thought so for a considerable period of time. Erickson, even though he had never met the patient before, was able to utilize this belief to bring about a major and rapid shift in the patient's life. He walked up to the patient on a hospital ward and said, "I heard you used to be a carpenter." Of course he got an affirmative reply. He then said, "And I heard you like to help people." Again the patient was required by his belief system to give an affirmative reply. Erickson said, "Good. Here's the hammer. They'll be doing construction out on the West Wing. I'd like you to go out and help them." The patient was soon engaged in "occupational therapy," something that he had refused to do previously. Shortly thereafter the patient was able to go home, simply because he had been working in an environment with a group of hard-hats who were not about to discuss with him the merits of whether he was or wasn't the Son of God. He had to learn to get along in the world without sharing his beliefs about who he was.

Another example of this principle demonstrating utilization of environment occurred when one of the authors was hypnotizing someone in his house. During the initial induction procedure, someone else in the house began to take a shower and the noise became quite intrusive. Rather than letting the noise become an interference, the author just continued with induction by saying, "and as you find yourself getting more relaxed you'll imagine warm water dripping down your back and with each drop you will find yourself getting more relaxed than previously." In this case the so-called intrusion became an auditory aid to the induction procedure.

Several more examples will be presented here to more clearly illustrate this important aid to effective communication.

A social worker was working with an alcoholic who exhibited an extreme need to be the center of attention (a symptom that often occurs with alcoholics). Rather than seeing this as another neurotic symptom that accompanied the alcoholism, the therapist was able to use this particular behavior as the way of treating the alcoholism. He simply began talking to the person about people he knew who gave up alcohol and how much attention they got because everyone knew how hard it was for an alcoholic to stop drinking; once they were able to do that, they were able to really brag and become the center of attention with their friends. This was an effective strategy in that the alcoholic finally found some reason that was good *for him* to give up alcohol.

A physical therapist was working with a farmer who had been making steady progress after a knee operation, but who was very dissatisfied with the slowness of his progress. Since the therapist knew that this person already had an understanding of farming, he simply began to draw analogies between the progress of the knee and the progress of the plant. He explained that if you looked every day at the plant you become very frustrated because the progress is very slow, and yet if you looked every few weeks or every month and measured progress that way, you could see the plant begin to sprout, begin to flower, and become a full-fledged healthy plant. This farmer was able to use his understanding of nature as a way of appreciating the progress he made, even if the speed was not what he originally would have liked.

An occupational therapist was working with a young male teenager who had lost the use of a hand. The teenager seemed uninterested in doing the hard work required to learn a new skill and during the training sessions was more interested in talking about football, his primary interest in life. The occupational therapist set up a scoreboard of progress. Every time the patient tried a task but didn't do very well, the therapist would take a towel out of her pocket and throw it down, symbolizing a penalty flag. On the other hand, every time the client did exceptionally well in learning a new task, the therapist would whistle, raise her hands to symbolize a touchdown, and put up seven points on the scoreboard. This is another example of utilizing a particular interest in a person's life and molding that interest toward the therapeutic goal desired.

One night, one of the authors was awakened at 3 A.M. by the intern in the emergency room to see a hysterical patient who said that his legs were totally paralyzed. A year before, the author would have come downstairs venting much anger and frustration (and four-letter words), dwelling on why things like that only happened when he was on call, why this guy had to pick this particular hospital to come to, and so on. Instead, the author found himself rushing downstairs, thinking, "What a fun opportunity this will be." As he entered the room the patient was just then saying that he was experiencing severe cramps in his left leg, while his right leg was still paralyzed and numb. Without hesitation, the author immediately utilized this piece of information, congruently saying, "That's wonderful, the cramps mean that the muscle strength is beginning to come back and will continue to return in the next few minutes—no doubt before long you'll also feel cramps in your right leg." Within one minute, cramps were also present in that leg, and five minutes later he was walking around the room testing his new found strength.

An occupational therapist's elderly patient had refused to participate in her A.D.L. (Activities of Daily Living) program because she said that she was too weak to even stand in the kitchen, let alone to do chores. With the knowledge that the patient was in the hospital for a stroke and had achieved a good recovery of her neurological functioning, the therapist suggested the weakness was more functional than organic. Instead of challenging the patient, however, she utilized the "weakness" and said, "Good, since you *are* so weak and since you will obviously need to get along by yourself in your house, what you need to do is build a stool that will support you while you're cooking and washing." The patient readily agreed, and after proudly finishing her chair one week later had regained most of her strength.

A child development specialist was asked by a school system to recommend

year-old girl. This second grader had an I.Q. of over 160
_elfth grade level. However, she was hostile to adults and
_dge about how to play or interact with children her own age.
_s severely overweight. The parents were both very bright profes-
sic _ople—the father was a well-known scientist and the mother was a
readıng specialist for a private school in the area. The child development
professional believed that the child needed a play therapy program but knew
that the parents (who thought that the daughter's only problem was boredom
in school) would never consent to treatment. The specialist noticed two
consistent patterns in the parents' behavior that proved to be critical in the
treatment process. First, it became clear that the mother made all the decisions
in the family. The father was nearly as socially unskilled as his daughter.
Second, the mother was a social snob. Among other things, the family dressed
in nothing but the most expensive clothes, and the mother would not let the
child play with other children in the neighborhood because "they weren't the
right kind." Both one-person domination of a family unit and social snobbery
can be seen as pathologic behaviors; however, given the principle of utilization
of behavior, they can also be seen as a gift given to the specialist to aid in the
treatment. Parental permission was obtained for the girl to be placed in the
much needed play therapy because the professional approached the mother
with the following invitation: "There is a new child therapist in town with a
national reputation who is only taking a limited number of cases. I've talked
to him, and because your daughter is so gifted and interesting and also because
her problems are so relatively minor, he has consented to take her on if you
wish."

A nursing student who had just attended a seminar given by the authors
was confronted with a patient who refused to take a laxative prescribed for
him. The observant nurse remembered that during the past few days the
patient had commented a number of times as to how good-humored a fellow
he was. Also, during a previous conversation that day, he had told the nurse
that he considered himself a good sport. The nurse asked him if he knew
which was his left hand and which was his right. When he smiled and said
yes, the nurse asked, "Will you take this medicine if I can show you that you
don't?" Of course the patient said yes. The nurse pointed to his left hand and
said, "Put this behind your back." She then asked, "Which one is left?" The
patient first smiled, then laughed, then drank his laxative. The patient was
clearly a good sport and the nurse was an effective communicator.

PERCEIVING THINGS IN A DIFFERENT WAY

We would like to conclude this chapter by presenting three more strategies for
more effective communication. The first of these is that we ourselves always
remember, and we work hard to get our clients to understand, that no matter
how you look at the world, there are always alternative ways to do so. Some
of these alternatives may be more helpful than the client's current view when
they begin treatment. Even though the authors see very different kinds of

patients in many different settings, they often find it useful to tell a story similar to the following:

> You know, I have a friend and his name is Bob. And Bob just got married and he was telling me recently that his in-laws are very inconsiderate people and that he's having a lot of problems with them. He said that of all the inconsiderate things they do, the most inconsiderate, the most irritating to him, was that they often come to his house unannounced. He told me that it was getting to the point that he dreaded being home because even when they weren't there he kept thinking that any minute they might arrive. This went on until one day when the doorbell rang; he opened the door, and it was then that he had the following insight: He realized that now that they were here, that meant that it was only going to be a relatively short time until they left and wouldn't be back again for a period of time. (Originally told by Joseph Barber)

This story was originally told to someone with chronic pain from a cancerous tumor who complained that the biggest problem she had was not only dealing with the pain when it was there, but anticipating the pain she knew would return even when it wasn't there. The message and implication of the story go far beyond the treatment of the particular symptom for which it was developed.

Getting the Patient to Act

Another effective communication strategy that helps patients see themselves as active agents in the treatment process is the strategy of having the clients *do* something regularly. By this we mean that it is important that the client actually do some activity other than just showing up for the appointment or taking a few pills. When we went to visit Milton Erickson, we found ourselves getting up early in the morning and climbing a 6,000-foot mountain to watch the sunrise. We later realized that Erickson had us do this not because he believed there was anything on top of the mountain relevant to what we came to talk to him about (or was there?), but rather that it was important for us, as part of the learning process, to understand that we were active agents—that we did not come just to listen passively to Milton Erickson tell stories. This strategy also introduces an element of control in that if the health professional can get the patient to do something that does not seem relevant to the treatment, it produces a mind set wherein the patient will cooperate with the health professional.

Issues of Power and Control

The issue of control in the treatment process is a very complex one. We believe that for people to be able to be active agents of change, they need to have an element of control over the situation. Just as no teacher can be effective unless he or she has some control over the classroom, no health professional can be effective without some control over the therapeutic situation. Yet it is also important for clients to feel as if they also have control over their own life (which, of course, they do). That is why throughout the book we stress techniques that give the health professional control, yet do it in such a way that the client believes that he is in control and consequently the dyad can work in *cooperation*. For example, in Chapter 6 we will be talking about a method that we call illusion of choice. By this method, health professionals always get the outcome they desire, but in a way that allows patients to make many choices; patients end up feeling in control and feeling good about themselves.

Control and power are two issues that many schools in the health professions deal with only implicitly. Many of the health professions take extreme views of these issues. Schools of counseling, for example, often teach that it is bad for health professionals to have any type of control and that their only goal is to give to clients a feeling of being in control of their life. This is a simplistic view of the clients' problems, a view that is not necessarily helpful in changing the clients' or patients' symptoms. At the other extreme are many medical schools that do not ever help physicians to learn methods to help their patients to feel somewhat in control. This is why many people feel alienated or in a childlike position when leaving the physician's office, as if they have just talked to a parent.

Humor

One of the most effective therapeutic strategies that we know of is the use of humor. Most people in this world today take themselves and their situations too seriously. This is especially true of people who are hurting and who come to a health professional. While at one level it is important to take each patient seriously, it is also important to help the patient understand the meaning of Humphrey Bogart's quote at the end of *Casablanca*: "In this crazy world the problems of three people don't amount to a hill of beans."

As mentioned before, the ideas and attitudes that most of us in the health professions have about "professionalization" are dysfunctional to treatment because they require us to take ourselves and our positions very seriously. Therefore, our patients can't help doing the same thing for themselves and their disorders. The most effective therapeutic use of humor is for the health professional to make fun of himself or herself. By not taking yourself so seriously you model to the client this concept and they learn not to take themselves so seriously. One of the authors, who is a psychologist, usually starts a formal conference presentation or a guest lecture to a new class with the following story:

> There was a seven-year-old boy named Billy in the second grade and one day Billy came to school going like this (the author holds his cupped hands in front of him, moving them around). The teacher said, "What are you doing Billy?" and Billy said, "Molding." The teacher said, "And what are your molding with?" and Billy said, "Shit." And the teacher said, "What are you molding?" and Billy said, "A teacher." So the teacher sent Billy to the principal's office and Billy walked into the principal's office repeating his hand gestures. The principal said, "What are you doing?" Billy said, "Molding." The principal said, "What are you molding

with?" Billy said, "Shit." The principal said, "What are you molding?" and Billy said, "A principal." So the principal does the ultimate thing; he sends Billy to the school psychologist's office, and the psychologist says, "Hey Billy, I bet you're molding." Billy shakes his head yes. He said, "Hey Billy, I bet you're molding with shit." Billy shakes his head yes. He said, "Hey Billy, I bet you're molding a psychologist." And Billy opens up his hands and looks and shakes his head no and says, "Not enough shit."

This story never fails to loosen up the audience and get its attention. It also puts the presentation in a certain perspective that says, "Okay, we are going to work here. The world's not going to end by what we do here, so let's relax and enjoy learning." Within this climate of relaxation and humor, inidividual problems often do not seem as heavy and powerful, allowing change to become easier. The idea that learning can be enjoyable is a strategy that most teachers never use. They wonder why their students don't enjoy coming to class or don't remember the material very long past the previous test.

We would like to re-emphasize the importance of the impact of the clients' belief system (or what we call reality) on their behavior. We do so by remembering an event involving an athlete who is now a well-known physician. It was believed for a long time that it was not possible for a human to run a mile under four minutes. Though athletes trained hard and many approached the mark, no one was able to run that mile under four minutes. One day Roger Bannister broke the four-minute mile, and very shortly afterwards many people were breaking it because it was suddenly believed that it was possible to run a mile under four minutes. Likewise, your belief system and your patient's belief system are incredibly important factors in the course and outcome of any treatment process.

EXERCISES

1. List and discuss important *reality strategies* associated with your profession. How do these strategies or beliefs affect patient care and treatment? Which strategies or beliefs do you think should be eliminated or modified to enhance treatment effectiveness? What new strategies or beliefs do you think should be added?
2. Sit opposite a partner. Notice your judgment about the other person's physical features, personality, and clothing. Begin to be aware of where these evaluations came from. Discuss.
3. Identify a difficult patient that you are working with or that you know. Now, keeping the concept of utilization of behavior in mind, devise a therapeutic plan (or some effective communication pattern) that would make use of that patient's characteristics or symptoms.

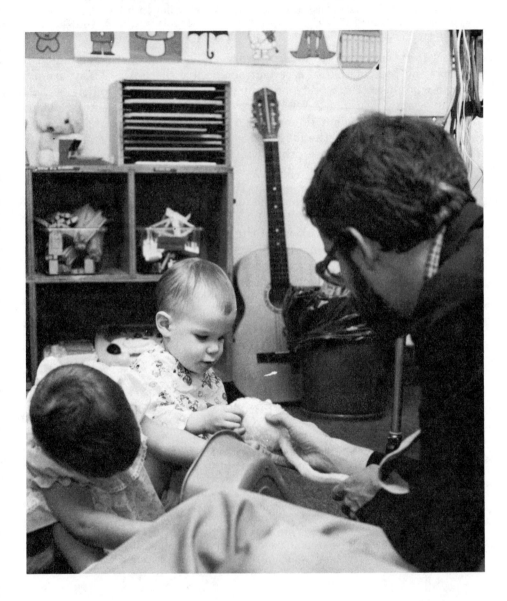

Pacing the Client's World 2

The first specific strategy of effective communication that we will discuss is pacing. The health professional will probably find pacing to be one of the most powerful techniques and yet one of the easiest to master. As you read about communications strategies in this chapter as well as in future chapters, we expect that you will recall examples of your own patterns of communication that parallel these and will be able to expand on them naturally.

As you sit there reading this sentence, noticing the color and texture of the page and the position of your forearms, you begin to be aware of the temperature of the room . . . the rhythm of your breathing . . . the pauses in your breathing now . . . you become increasingly aware of the sounds and slight noises around you. This is an example of pacing. In pacing, the communicator begins by presenting to a person a statement or statements that are immediately verifiable by that person's experience. As this is being done, an instant and ongoing rapport with the subject is being established. In this way, suggestions or other messages can be offered with a higher probability of acceptance. Though it may seem overly simple (and you're right—it is!), the whole idea of effective communication can be summarized as an interplay between pacing and leading, the latter referring to the suggestions offered when and only when the former has been accomplished adequately.

A review of the previous example should help to make this phenomenon more clear. Since you were all obviously looking at the page when you started reading the paragraph, beginning the statement with "As you sit there reading this sentence . . ." ensures that what we begin with is a statement that matches your experience at that moment. We are not suggesting that after reading this you consciously thought to yourself that indeed this is what was happening. In fact, quite the contrary—there was a level of experience below your level of awareness that agreed with what you were reading. Note the different feeling you get if we started with "As you sit there reading aloud this sentence. . . ." For most of you, that would be an inadequate pace.

Continuing with the example, we next mention your awareness of seeing the page, its color and texture. This is actually a lead phrase, but one that was

19

an easy jump from the preceding one. This phrase in turn leads you to become aware of the position of your forearms. This process continues until you are led to an awareness of the sounds around you. In the same manner, the last statement can then be incorporated into the pace for further leading. The stronger the pace becomes, the greater the likelihood that subsequent suggestions will be accepted.

VERBAL PACING

Although the order of statements in the above example was somewhat important, this need not always be the case. One can simply mention to a person several statements with which he or she will agree. Thus if a child has just abraded a knee from a fall, a few appropriate statements such as the following could be immediately offered: "I bet that hurts terribly," "It's even starting to bleed a little," "No wonder you're crying, I'd be screaming too." Phrases such as these, spoken congruently with the appropriate expression and feeling, but not in any particular order, would usually establish an adequate pace for the child at that moment. Inserting a lead statement such as, "And I bet that will *continue* to really hurt terribly, maybe for a whole minute or two," usually results in the desired outcome—the cessation of pain in a minute or two. Contrast this approach with a more typical approach one might almost instinctively take with such a child; that is, to say "It doesn't hurt that much" (almost trying to convince the child that his or her experience of pain is not valid). Since there is no congruence between your verbalized expression and the child's experience, you have not set up the conditions necessary to lead the child out of the pain.

Another example of effective pacing and leading is illustrated by the following. One of the authors was paged to the emergency room in the early morning hours to see a woman in her late fifties who was insisting on admission to the hospital. The intern on duty had carefully reviewed her records and noted that she had just been discharged. A psychosomatic process had been diagnosed several weeks previously. She now complained of the same symptoms. Leafing through all of the x-ray studies and lab tests confirmed the diagnosis in the intern's mind. After performing a physical examination, which had negative results, the intern concluded that the patient's symptoms suggested the same functional process and that the woman should be discharged from the ER to follow up with her local doctor the next morning. He repeatedly explained the situation in a reasonable and patient manner to the woman. She kept insisting that she was too weak to survive returning home and that there definitely *was* something very real wrong with her. This ping-pong game continued until the intern in exasperation called for the author's assistance.

Now let's break for a moment and, in typical sportscaster fashion, analyze the match so far. The intern, playing with his Sprague Rappaport aluminum stethoscope and clad in white coat and matching tennis shoes, carries with him his superior intellectual reasoning and impressive medical jargon. The patient, though lacking in accoutrements, realizes that this may be her last appearance and is ready to give it all she's got. This latter point should be emphasized and, in fact, compassionately understood, since in her view of her world at that moment, she was in a dangerous state of health and didn't know whether or not she would survive through the night.

Continuing the metaphor, as the game continues in a deadlock, the important principle of requisite variety, discussed in Chapter 1, can now be exercised. The principle states that if you try something and it does not work, try something else rather than endlessly repeating the ineffective communication.

After reviewing the records and getting a brief summary from the intern, including what had already been told to the patient, the author walked into the patient's room. She appeared generally anxious, but not in pain. After examining her, the author said, "Obviously, there is something definitely wrong with you that we failed to pick up on the last admission. Why else would you feel as weak and tired as you do?" From the relieved look on her face it was apparent that this was the first time that night that she had found someone who knew something and whom she could trust. With a few sentences, the author established a rapport upon which to build. Furthermore, she was not being lied to because she obviously had a disorder that needed attention. After repeating the previous statements in different words and again noting from her facial relaxation, nods, and appreciative replies that she was adequately paced, it was a simple feat to lead her around the next lap. The author said, "Since we both agree that there is something wrong that needs to be discovered, we have one of two options. We can bring you back in the hospital to repeat the same tests; that is, drawing your blood twice a day and having you lie on the x-ray tables for more pictures." Her horizontal head shaking at that point indicated that the intervention was on the right track. "Or else we can take some definite action with your doctor in the morning and schedule some new lines of investigation." She liked this idea much more and after working out some small details concerning transportation, she went home.

Another beautiful example of pacing and leading was demonstrated by a music therapist who was working as the music director in a summer camp for mentally retarded teenagers and adults. One day she noticed a young woman with a history of withdrawal and depression leaving her music session crying and whining. The therapist walked up to her (knowing she was trying to learn to play the recorder) and said, "You're not feeling very good now, are you?" The camper said, "No, my thumbs just will not stay on the holes." The music director then said, "I had the same trouble when I was learning to play the recorder. Do you know what I did?" The camper looked up very curiously and shook her head. The therapist said, "First I yelled at my thumbs. I said, 'Thumbs! Why don't you stay on those holes!' You know what?" When the camper shook her head no, the therapist said, "My thumbs just weren't very scared of me and didn't respond to my yelling." She then said, "So you know what I did next?" And after the appropriate pause and noticing from the wide-eyed stare of the camper that she was clearly curious and her attention had been secured, the therapist said, "I started crying and whining, 'Thumbs, why don't you ever do the right thing?' And you know what?" Again, waiting until the camper shook her head no, she said, "My thumbs just didn't have any sympathy with my whining and crying." The therapist looked at her, seeing that clearly an adequate pace had been established, and realized that she could lead her on to the next step. "So I said to my thumbs, 'Okay, I know you'll do it whenever you're ready and I'm just going to keep practicing and wait to see when you're able to stay over the holes.' " She then told the camper, "Besides, there's no right or wrong way to do this, the fun thing about music is to just experiment." She reported that the camper broke into a smile and walked away. The next day at the music lesson, as the therapist walked by the session she heard the camper saying to her individual counselor, "Oh, hi! I'm just experimenting until my thumbs get ready."

To repeat, for a health professional, nothing takes the place of adequate training or experience in his or her field. However, adequate training and experience still may not be very helpful to your patients if you are not able to communicate effectively with them.

NONVERBAL PACING

Thus far in this chapter we have been discussing one aspect of pacing, namely verbal pacing. As previously described, the process involves meeting patients in their view of the world through language. Only after accepting their models of reality can we hope to move from there. Another equally powerful type of pacing is nonverbal pacing. (A detailed discussion of nonverbal communication skills will be presented in Chapter 5.) In using nonverbal pacing, various aspects of a person's body language are mirrored, including rate of breathing, body posture, hand and arm movement and voice tone, tempo, and amplitude. In this approach, the communicator chooses one or several of these components and in a subtle manner mimics them during the interaction. This is naturally often done simultaneously with verbal pacing, but, as will be shown, that is not necessary. This technique may at first seem very arduous, even silly. However, several clarifications, followed by examples, should demonstrate to you how this can be easily mastered. Nonverbal pacing is a profoundly powerful mechanism in helping to secure the appropriate groundwork needed for successful communication and especially for the establishment of trust.

As in verbal pacing, it is not necessary that all of the body language be mirrored. Specifically, if a patient is talking very rapidly, one can choose to pace the rate of speech without also mimicking the fast breathing and hand movements. Or if a patient is slouching way down in a chair, just the posture can be copied. For example, talking to a child in an unfamiliar environment is greatly facilitated by stooping down so that eye levels are parallel.

A particularly noteworthy example of this technique occurred at a conference in Philadelphia sponsored by the Temple University Department of Psychiatry. Frank Farrelly, a nationally recognized psychotherapist, was conducting a model therapy session in front of about 500 people with a client picked from the audience. While it would be reasonable to assume that it might be difficult to achieve any degree of significant interaction in front of all of those people, this is exactly what happened. The client afterwards said that he had felt deeply and securely enmeshed in the interaction; in fact, he said he had felt "stoned." Though Dr. Farrelly is known to transmit that degree of security and trust to his clients, when queried he was not able to say exactly what it was he did that was responsible for the results. Richard Bandler and John Grinder, who had observed the session, noted some very specific behaviors. When Dr. Farrelly sat down with the client, he assumed an almost identical posture—in this case, slumping back with his knees crossed. Within one minute, Dr. Farrelly was breathing at exactly the same rate as the client and continued this throughout the session. Interestingly, although below the conscious awareness of Dr. Farrelly (as well as that of the patient), these unconscious nonverbal strategies were extremely effective in contributing to a profoundly rich and trusting therapeutic relationship.

Just as this talented therapist was not consciously using these techniques, most of us are unaware that we display many of the same behaviors in our interactions with patients, family, and friends. Look at your own verbal patterns and notice how many times you start a reply with a phrase such as, "Yes, I can understand that you must be very frustrated with this situation," or, "I agree that you look tired; you put in a hard day yesterday." From such statements you often continue in a natural fashion with lead phrases. Unconscious nonverbal pacing in our behavior is just as common. When a person speaks fast and loudly to us, or slowly and softly, we tend to respond at the same level.

As an exercise, for two to three minutes a day, observe couples talking to each other. Stay far enough away so that it is not obvious that you are watching. Aim your eyes at a spot directly between both people. Let your eyes defocus from that spot and you will easily be able to see both people's movements simultaneously. You will begin to observe how people lean forward at the same time, move their hands in similar fashion, and so on. Also listen to the tonal patterns of their speech. This is easiest if you ignore the content of their conversation, but listen instead to the form; i.e., the tempo, timbre, and amplitude. Notice again how these patterns parallel each other. As you do this exercise, you will experientially learn how we are all to varying degrees continually utilizing both types of pacing. The same can be said for all of the techniques that will be discussed in this book. Our goal is for you to bring these patterns to a level of total conscious awareness so that you can utilize them more often and more effectively in appropriate interactions.

A good way to learn nonverbal pacing is to practice one aspect of it at a time. Thus at first, you may decide to assume a similar posture to a patient (or friend). This does not mean mimicking the exact same position, but holding the shoulders, arms, legs, and face in mirror-like fashion. Later you can practice with breathing rate, gesture, and voice tone. Although each of these may at first seem to require supreme mental effort and concentration (thinking of it as a game helps a lot!), soon this new technique will become so automatic that you will be able to perform it unconsciously, without any effort at all. At first, learning to drive a car requires a lot of work and concentration. After a while, we leave the driving mostly to our unconscious, as our conscious minds are more concerned with the day's events, our next meal, and various daydreams that we are busy creating.

KEEP PACING BELOW CONSCIOUS AWARENESS

Another consideration of paramount importance is that the pacing must be kept below the client's conscious awareness. If you keep repeating exactly what someone is saying to you, the person will soon realize what you are doing. In the same way, if you overtly mimic aspects of the patient's body language, this too will easily be noticed, thereby losing its intended effect. Incidentally, this is why matching the patient's breathing pattern is so effective—it is virtually always below the patient's conscious awareness.* Often a person will withdraw abruptly from a particular posture if that position is overtly mirrored. Find someone in an unusual pose—i.e., hand on head, leaning way over in a chair—and assume that exact position. You'll be able to see the immediate reflex withdrawal. You might recall that in the first example of this chapter, when the rhythm of your breathing was called to your awareness, you had the paradoxical reaction of pausing for a minute. We therefore incorporated the pausing directly into the overall pace. Again, the main idea is to keep the pacing at a level that can be unconsciously appreciated. This manifests itself in a heightened degree of trust and rapport, rather than in a self-conscious withdrawal.

A striking example of nonverbal pacing occurred in a New York City high school several years ago. A teacher whose particularly unruly class had often left him powerless in controlling their behavior, had left the room for several minutes. Upon returning, he found the students engaged in what looked and sounded like a drunken debacle—students standing on desks, yelling, fighting, and making animal sounds. Perhaps the outlandishness of the situation was enough to produce the requisite variety needed. Instead of pleading and reasoning with the class as he had done in the past, he simply shouted out in an extremely loud, raucous voice, "Let's have some pandemonium here!" Despite his contradictory verbal message, the tone of his voice had adequately paced the overall insanity of the room. The class fell silent immediately.

CONGRUENCE

In making the distinction between verbal and nonverbal pacing, it has some-times been assumed that with the former strategy only the actual words that

---

*Breathing at the same rate as another is only one example of this. Another excellent choice is to match the cadence of your own talking to someone else's breathing, so that the beginning of every small phrase or group of words matches each inspiration or expiration.

the communicator utters are important. We would like to emphasize again that any communication, if it is to be effective, must be accompanied by the appropriate body language. In the previous example concerning the woman in the emergency room, if the author involved had stood there telling her in monotones that she was sick and really did need further tests, while at the same time rolling his eyes upward as if asking the Lord why he had picked that night to send in this crazy person, the effect would have been entirely different. Thus, successful communication involves congruence, or making one's body language consistent with the verbalization that is offered. In everyday terms, talking congruently is usually perceived by us as talking sincerely, earnestly, or with a lot of expression. In essence, when we hear and see a congruent message, we get the inexpressible feeling that the person is speaking the truth. When you think of particular instances in which you felt someone was talking sincerely, you realize that, besides the content of what he or she was saying, your unconscious awareness of body movement and voice tonality is what produced this feeling. If, while congruently pacing people verbally, you add to this a subtle mirroring of certain aspects of their body language by your own, you have then incorporated nonverbal pacing into your behavior as well.

A subject akin to communicator congruence is patient congruence. When a physical therapy outpatient glances down at the floor and stiffly brings his arm up, scratching the side of his head as he tells his therapist that he did indeed do his exercises that week, the therapist may get an intuitive uneasy feeling as to whether or not what the patient said was true. Certain police departments, in fact, have listed specific body movements—such as shifting of eyes downward and shuffling of feet—as signals to an interrogating officer that a suspect or witness may be lying. As we begin to learn to SEE AND HEAR PATIENTS MORE CLEARLY, we will begin to make these distinctions more sharply. A major advantage of close observation is being able to notice when a person has different parts of himself or herself that have conflicting views or feelings on a particular subject. The patient who says that she is not scared of her upcoming surgery, while at the same time starting to breathe more shallowly and rapidly, is often not lying. Part of her knows that it will be a simple surgical case with a low incidence of complications. Another part remembers a friend who died 8 years ago of a similar "simple" surgery.

The preceding example is not an unusual one. The people whom health professionals deal with are often in a state of anxiety. One typical response to such a state is to develop ambivalent feelings about one's self and one's situation. There is a part of each patient that wants to be rational and mature and to believe that only good can happen. There is also a scared little kid in each patient. When health professionals ask a patient before a procedure if he feels okay and the patient says yes but shakes his head slightly in a negative direction or has a lump in the throat, rather than ignoring such nonverbal information and acting as if things were okay (which does not pace part of the patient's feelings), one could say, "I guess you have mixed feelings because part of you wants to feel okay while the lump in your throat indicates that you are still scared. How can I help you feel better?'' The most important outcome of such a conversation is not the immediate relief of the patient's fears (even though that might well happen), but rather that the health professional becomes one who knows and who cares and who can be trusted. The groundwork for a strong professional-patient relationship has been laid, along with a high probability of patient compliance.

CASE EXAMPLES

The following case illustrates an example of combining verbal and nonverbal pacing. In the early morning hours, the shift supervisor of nursing at a large Pittsburgh hospital was walking by the intensive care unit when she heard a loud argument. The intern and nurses reported that a patient was threatening that if he wasn't allowed to smoke a cigarette, he would leave. This patient, who had a history of cardiac and psychiatric disease, had several hours previously been a visitor at his wife's bedside in another section of the hospital. As he was leaving, he suddenly experienced severe substernal chest pain followed by a syncopal episode. He was immediately rushed to the ICU with a presumptive diagnosis of myocardial infarction. Naturally, strict bed rest is routinely prescribed, as is no smoking, because of the oxygen equipment. The staff had been trying to calm him for some time, but he continued to insist in a highly agitated manner that he wanted to smoke. After arriving and getting a summary, the nurse marched quickly into the room. She immediately began to speak in a loud, fast, and somewhat high-pitched and "agitated" voice. The staff, expecting soft, soothing tones and perhaps a lullaby or two, looked on in amazement. In the tone described and with the appropriate congruent body movement, such as exaggerated hand movements and moderately fast breathing, she proceeded to tell him, 'Of course you're upset. You've got severe pain. You're closed in here. Your wife's in the hospital, and on top of that they won't even let you relax a little by smoking one lousy cigarette. Boy, I'd be upset too. It's a wonder you've been able to tolerate it as long as you have.'' Having his complete attention, she continued in this fashion for several minutes while very carefully changing from pacing to leading. Specifically, she very gradually began to slow down and soften her speech and breathe slower and move more smoothly. Within about five minutes, she noticed that, although he was beginning to relax, a couple of times he started to momentarily get a little more agitated. Having the sensory experience to notice as soon as this happened, she modulated her behavior back upwards to again adequately pace his own. When she was satisfied again that she was pacing him, she would return to leading toward relaxation. Within about seven minutes, he was calm, having only occasional episodes of pain that agitated him momentarily. At this point, he actually looked up at her and said, "You know, for some reason I really think I can trust you." With this rapport established, it was a simple matter to arrange a deal with him concerning when he could next smoke. The patient's case was then privately discussed among the nurses and resident on duty, and they agreed that they would use the same strategy if the behavior recurred that night. It didn't, but one of the nurses present told the authors that several weeks later she used the same technique effectively on an agitated post-surgical patient.

The ideas that we are describing and the ones that will be found in future chapters have all been demonstrated to be very effective forms of communication. It is important to acknowledge, however, that we are not suggesting that these are the only valuable communication methods. There are as many ways to say something as there are words in our vocabulary. The governing principle is whether or not what you are communicating is achieving the desired outcome with a specific patient at a specific time. If the answer is yes, continue to practice what you're doing, using our suggested techniques simply for interest or variation. If, as with most of us, a significant percentage of patients with whom you communicate are not reached satisfactorily, a dramatic increase in your effectiveness will start with your having the adequate sensory experience to notice it—whether you do so immediately or within the next day or week. A willingness to try out these new strategies, even if they seem a bit awkward at first, will no doubt result in equipping you with the extra tools needed to make a significant difference in your overall effectiveness as a health professional.

This idea is clearly exemplified by a dentist with whom we recently talked. He said that when new patients who seem scared enter his office, he simply talks slowly and in a soft, but firm voice, while looking as relaxed as he can. He talks about what he is going to do and deliberately ignores their fear. Since the experience is usually free of significant pain, patients have little difficulty after the initial session. This strategy works well for him and his patients most of the time. However, with a small percentage of patients this technique simply does not work adequately. Some patients sit trembling in their chairs for the whole session, often reacting very strongly to any pressure sensation in even well-anesthetized areas. A couple of clients have walked out before work was started because of intense fear. Thus his style in this subset of patients was not working satisfactorily. The ones who stayed proved very tedious to work with—not to mention the terror they experienced during the hour.

At this point, he agreed to experiment with some of these techniques, beginning with pacing. With his next tense patient, he said, "I can see that you're kind of nervous; you just look like I feel when I visit my family doctor. No matter what he says, I'm still frightfully nervous for the first five or ten minutes until he is in the middle of examining me, when I finally begin to realize that IT'S MUCH MORE COMFORTABLE THAN I IMAGINED POSSIBLE." Of course, he said the whole thing congruently, but without the use of nonverbal pacing at first. As he became comfortable with this, he then began to add nonverbal elements—specifically, matching the rhythm of his talking with the patient's breathing and mirroring shoulder position. After one or two minutes, he would gradually begin to slow his voice down and lower his shoulders. Six weeks later, he found a great increase in the total number of patients with whom he could work smoothly.

What we have said so far can probably best be summarized with a six-word sentence uttered one day by an occupational therapist in a private mental hospital. This statement fully represents combination of pacing and leading, in both verbal and nonverbal aspects. A patient had stationed himself inside a room, screaming, cursing, and disrupting the furniture. Initial efforts by the staff could not stop him. The therapist, who was passing by, walked in and yelled in a loud, frantic voice, "YOU ARE REALLY UPSET!" After a two second pause the therapist continued in a slow, soft, soothing tone, with relaxed body accompaniment, *"weren't* you?" The patient answered in a clear, calm voice, as if the event had occurred the day before, that indeed he had been upset, and started to discuss the situation matter-of-factly with this staff member. In only a few moments this professional communicator was able to pace the patient's emotional state and lead him to an alternative state, thereby beginning the therapeutic process.

Many of the techniques to be discussed in the rest of the text are means of leading patients towards therapeutic goals consistent with your profession. Leading patients is a difficult task unless you can first pace the clients' understanding of the world and their ways of behaving in it. When you do learn to pace clients, you will find that leading becomes much easier because you have established a trusting relationship, often at a deeply unconscious level. Because pacing is so critical to the rest of the text, we will be returning to these ideas often. Another very powerful area of pacing utilizes representational systems. This subject and its clinical applications will be discussed in the next chapter.

EXERCISES

1. Give examples of past interactions with patients or other people in your life where pacing might have led to a more fruitful outcome.
2. Have one person make up a problem or symptom that is just a little bit exaggerated. The partner verbally paces what the narrator is saying and then finally takes the lead to any desired outcome.
3. Observe pairs or small groups of people for evidence of pacing or lack of it. Notice how people who are *really* communicating naturally end up pacing each others' speech and behavior.
4. While pacing a partner, have one person begin to talk about some subject or incident. The other's job is to nonverbally pace the narrator. Discuss the experience afterwards.
5. Practice another type of verbal pacing in which your partner's body language is verbally paced by you. Verbally state everything that you notice to be true about your partner's

nonverbal behavior. Thus, as he or she is breathing in, you say, "You are breathing in." Also pace things such as eye blinking, muscle twitching, and body shifting. Be sure to pace only things that you see, rather than what you guess. An example of what you see would be, "You're moving your left arm." An example of guessing would be, "You have a pain in your back," or "Your mind is beginning to wander." Discuss the experience afterwards.

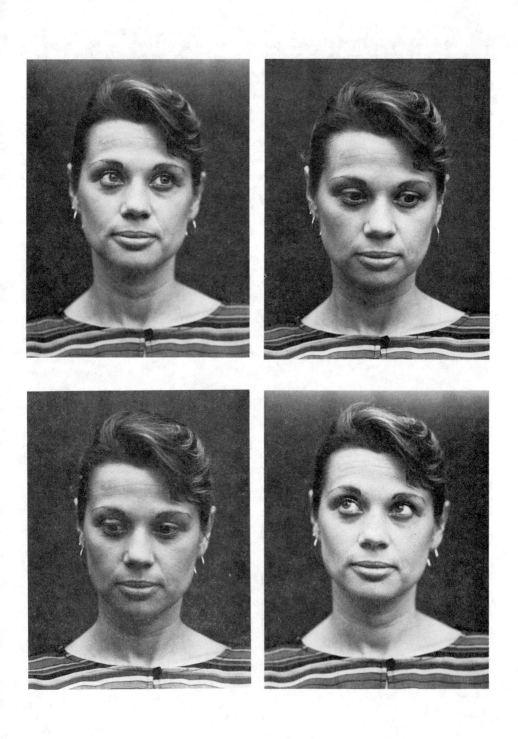

Representational 3
Systems

The waitress approaches as you sit comfortably in the booth, wiping the last red traces of your Burger Deluxe from your chin. She asks you if you'd like some dessert and you inquire as to the choices. Her head tilts to the left, and her eyes move up and left as she begins to recite the five selections. When she is done, you point with your index finger to a spot about two feet directly over her head and say, "I'll take that one." Her cheeks immediately become the previous color of your chin, as she reflexively covers her upper and lower torso with her hands. After she recovers, you smile and ask her what happened. She replies that she had the momentary feeling that you were seeing through her when you pointed to her dessert list like that, as if you had x-ray vision or something. You almost ask her if there's a nearby phone booth where you can don your red cape, but you reconsider and simply tell her, "I could see by your expression that you were visualizing that dessert list in your mind. When I pointed to what looked like a specific selection, you had the momentary feeling that I was seeing through you. You then immediately covered your body so that I couldn't see that too." She smiles and agrees that that is indeed what happened. You then say, "I've changed my mind, I'll take that one instead," pointing one foot over her head, "and incidentally, you have nice kidneys!"

As many of you are probably similarly unaware, most of you visualized that whole scene in your mind's eye as you were reading it; how much ketchup was on the customer's chin; whether the waitress was wearing a uniform or regular clothes; how big the restaurant was; which side of the table the customer was seated on. We all visualize internally whether or not we are consciously aware of it. This chapter is about the different ways in which people represent their experience and the techniques that enable us to distinguish one way from another for the purpose of communicating more effectively.

THE THREE SYSTEMS OF EXPERIENCING

If asked how you liked the beach the last time you were there, there would be several different ways in which each of you would answer. Some of you would get an internal visual picture and begin to describe the water, the graceful seagulls, or the shapes and bathing suits of people on the beach. Others might smile and begin to describe how soft the sand felt as you walked and lay on it, while feeling the satisfying warmth of the sun on your body and the cooling breeze from the water. Still others of you might predominantly describe the roar of the waves, the patter of feet running through the shallow water, and the laughter of little children scurrying from the oncoming waves. Actually we all remember aspects of each of these three modalities of visual, kinesthetic, and auditory phenomena. When we choose to experience data consciously— either while daydreaming or when communicating to others—we have a preferred dominant system by which we will represent that experience. We refer to this as a representational system. Thus, although there might (and probably would) be components of all three modalities in each of the descriptions, one of these would usually predominate. There are of course two other sensory modalities not yet mentioned by which we can represent our experience: taste and smell. While all of us organize some portion of our experience around these parameters, these are not preferred systems in our culture. We are, of course, different from a dog, who after visiting that same beach might choose to describe to its friends such things as the spicy aroma of the water, the pervasive smell of that stuff those people smeared all over their bodies, and the titillating scent of a particular poodle's bottom.

There are several ways of determining the preferred representational systems that a person is using. Two of the easiest ways are by watching eye scanning patterns and listening to the predicates that are used in sentences. After describing these two we will discuss their practical applicability, including their important relationship to the principles of pacing.

EYE SCANNING

There are consistent eye patterns that humans use when experiencing the different sensory modalities of visualization, kinesthetics, and audition. When most people form an internal image in their minds, their eyes turn up or point straight ahead with pupillary dilation. Recall when you've asked questions of friends or patients, and they have said "Hmm, let's see," as their eyes shifted up and to the left or right. Or when you're talking to others, you know that they're not looking at you, but at something far away. Most of us have a vague feeling, mainly at an unconscious level, when this is occurring. We also pick up on the relaxation of the facial muscles that accompanies pupillary dilation and the straight-ahead stare. Some of you might argue that you don't see all that stuff; however, you must admit that you can usually recognize and are aware when someone is in this dreamy type of state, even though you do not know that the person is actually seeing pictures. If you *are* aware of that state, then the information *must* be coming from somewhere. Assuming no assistance from "The Force" or other extraterrestrial powers, the clues must be arriving to you from your sensory experience.

If you are not yet convinced of your unconscious powers of observation, consider the following example. At a moment in time exactly five seconds before "now," most of you were not aware of the various background sounds around you, such as passing of outside cars, the wind against the window, and the ticking of the clock. If at any one second, however, any of these sounds had suddenly stopped, you would have consciously noticed the change. In order for us to notice a change in our environment, there needs to be at some level an awareness of what *was* going on. This awareness is often at the unconscious level. To understand the way that your patient currently represents his or her world and to make appropriate interventions requires that you as a health professional have a conscious knowledge of the representational system model.

There are two types of visual imagery that we all experience. One is eidetic imagery; the other, constructed imagery. Recall a time when you were on a roller coaster or similar ride and see yourself on it. . . . Now, instead, imagine that you're actually in the car and see the track ahead of you as you rush down the next slope. Notice the difference between the two scenes. Go ahead, we'll wait. . . . The first experience is called constructed imagery. None of you has really ever seen yourself sitting on a roller coaster before from another vantage point. In constructed imagery an image that has never been seen before is created in the mind's eye. Another example would be imagining a scene, such as a dinosaur walking on the street where you live or the President visiting your house for tea. When most right-handed people construct an image, their eyes will either shift up and to their right or point straight ahead with pupillary dilation, the latter also being called defocusing. The reason postulated for the upper right movement is that constructed imagery usually takes place in the dominant hemisphere. In almost all right-handed people and in most left-handers, pointing the eyes toward the right visual field correlates with left brain visualization activity. For each person these eye patterns are usually consistent over time. The bottom line is for you, the communicator, to notice in which direction a patient's eyes move when, for example, he tells you of his upcoming surgery the next morning. If he has not had the same operation performed before by the same surgeons, he will be constructing the image of himself lying on the operating table and seeing that image from a distance. If he is looking up and to his right during this time, you will know that this pattern will be consistent for him when he subsequently constructs other images. At a later date such information can be useful for effective communication.

Eidetic imagery, as demonstrated in the second part of the roller coaster example, is when you remember a scene as you saw it before. You no longer see yourself in the picture, only the things that your eyes actually saw at that time. With this type of imagery you are more likely to recover the original feelings and sounds of the previous experience. How many of you that had put yourself into the picture of the roller coaster were able to feel some of the fear or tightening up of your body or hear the sound of the iron wheels on the track build to a crescendo as the car raced down the slope. Eidetic imagery usually occurs in the nondominant hemisphere (usually the right); the eyes will therefore move up and to the left as this hemisphere is accessed. Again, this applies for most people and is consistent within each person. (Looking ahead with defocused eyes can also mean eidetic imagining, so that when someone is doing this all one can say is that he or she is visualizing.)

A nurse walking into a new patient's room with an injection might notice that the patient starts to breathe rapidly and in a shallow manner, while relating how bad the last experience was when receiving a shot. The nurse may notice that the person's eyes are up and to the left; thus, at that moment the nurse can guess that the patient is probably eidetically visualizing and recalling that last incident. Hence, at that exact moment in time, the nurse knows that the patient is experiencing lying in another place and watching another nurse or doctor coming up and administering an injection—and that the patient at that moment is experiencing the same fear that occurred previously. With this knowledge, the nurse can intervene in several ways at this stage, as will be discussed later in this chapter.

When most of us are recalling something kinesthetically, such as the feeling of the coldest day of last year, our eyes will move down and to the right. (For those who like mnemonics, an easy one here is "feels right.") Hearing something internally, like talking to oneself or creating the sound of a train, appears either as eyes shifting back and forth on a horizontal plane or looking down and to the left.

Actually, we do not want you to take our word as to the validity of these concepts, because we don't think that would be very useful. What would be particularly valuable (with this as well as with the other things that we talk about) is for you to go out and practice noticing these things in people whom you feel safe observing. This will verify in your own experience that these eye patterns do in fact exist and are consistent and at the same time will give you the practice needed to begin systematically noticing these patterns.

A good exercise involves sitting down with one or more people and asking them specific questions that you know will make them access either visual, kinesthetic, or auditory experiences. One or more people can be watching the eyes of the person being questioned. For instance, a visual question might be, "What was the color of your parents' last car?" or "What did your tenth grade math teacher look like?" Note that the question should not be too easy (like identifying the color of one's hair), since this is a fact that the person knows automatically and will not have to visualize in order to answer. Similarly, you can then ask a kinesthetic question like, "What does it feel like to stroke a horse's mane or to rub your feet on warm sand?" Asking the person to recall the sound of a passing fire truck or the singing of a nursery rhyme are examples of appropriate auditory questions.

When you first do these exercises and then observe them in patients, you'll need to be aware of one other phenomenon. If a person is asked to remember the feeling of the bark of a tree, for example, the *picture* of a certain tree may be recalled first. In visualizing the tree the person will then be able to describe feeling it. We call the former process the lead system—the sensory modality the person uses to bring things into consciousness. Observing this person's eyes, you'll probably see them go up and to the left at first and only then down and to the right. Thus, examining the eye scanning patterns lets you know system by system the sensory system that a person is experiencing at any moment. In this last example we know that a visual picture was created first, followed by a feeling. Similarly, if the question was to describe a new car, another person's eyes might have gone down and to the right for a moment and then up and to the left. Assuming this person was like the majority of right-handers, the lead system here was kinesthetic; in order to bring that information to consciousness he or she first had to experience the feeling of sitting in the driver's seat and then had to visualize the car. Thus, in our first example, the person's leading system was visual (seeing the tree), followed by a kinesthetic system (experiencing the feel of the bark). In the second example, this person's lead system was kinesthetic (feeling the new seat against his or her body), followed by visual (seeing the inside of the car).

When you start to notice these eye shifts, feel free to ask people what processes they went through in responding to your question. For instance, after asking someone the color of the first dress she could remember ever wearing, you might see her eyes dart up to the right, and then down to the right, followed again by the same sequence. You could then ask her if she saw herself as a child in a new dress and if she had a good feeling about that. She might affirm this and say that she pictured herself again, focusing on the color of the dress and experiencing a feeling of satisfaction about identification. Frequently, eye movements occur rapidly. So again, practice in identifying these patterns is emphasized.

PREDICATE USE

A second major way to be aware of representational systems is by listening to the specific predicates that people employ in their sentences. As mentioned in the preceding beach example, all of us have a sensory modality—whether visual, kinesthetic, or auditory—that we use more often than others when representing our experience. In relating this experience to others, we unconsciously choose words that are appropriate to our mode of thinking at that moment. Being able to systematically know what a person's preferred representational system is can be an important tool. We can use it to further our capabilities of meeting the patient in his or her model of the world. This can be done by modifying our own predicates to match the patient's system. In this way predicate use can be thought of as another tool of effective pacing. Consider how utilizing this could be useful in the following hypothetical discussion:

> Patient: I just don't feel I'm ready for an operation. It's hard for me to think of lying down on that cold table to be cut into.

Surgeon: Well, I want you to see that it's clearly necessary that we operate. You've got a fibroid the size of a grapefruit that's taking up a lot of space in there.

Patient: But I'm most scared about how bad I'll feel after surgery. It's hard for me to grasp how this fibroid can be so dangerous if it's benign. I just don't think I can handle surgery right now.

Surgeon: Okay. But I'm sure you can see that it's not going to get any smaller. Clearly this will have to come out. I hope you get the picture.

Patient: Yes, but I still don't feel good about it.

This is a rather blatant example of *mis*matching of representational systems between a surgeon and a patient. If you haven't picked up the clues, why not read it again.

The patient's representational system is kinesthetic. Notice the choice of predicates in the sentences—words like feel, hard, cold, cut, grasp, handle. These and other words, such as contact, come in touch with, and come to grips with, presuppose a kinesthetic experience. People whose representational system is predominantly kinesthetic organize their reality mostly around how things feel around them, how things fit into place, or how things match together. They do more things out of a general sense that something or other will feel right. This is not to say that they don't make decisions based on visual modes of thinking as well. It just means that they use their kinesthetic system most often.

Did you also pick up on the surgeon's predicates—clearly, see, get the picture. These and other words, such as vivid, bright, imagine, color, and looks like, imply a visual representational system. Notice that the example we have just given is quite different from our previous example of how different people would describe their experience at the beach. It is very easy to perceive if someone is talking about how good the sand felt or how pretty the sky was. In the surgery example, they were not talking about a topic described so easily in either terms exclusively. However, if you listen to the predicates (that is, verbs, adjectives, and adverbs), you can easily discover that the patient is organizing the experience in a primarily kinesthetic mode. Obviously the doctor is not being entirely effective in this situation. Though what the doctor is saying makes a lot of sense medically, the patient did not go to medical school and is experiencing many uneasy feelings about the operation. The doctor does have another choice, however, assuming that the doctor knows about representational systems or possesses an unconscious ability to match representational systems (like a lot of effective communicators do). The doctor can simply structure sentences to include kinesthetic predicates. For example, the doctor could acknowledge the patient's feelings of fear and reassure the patient that adequate anesthesia and pre-op and post-op medications will be given and that discomfort will be minimal. The doctor could explain how the mass is causing pressure on the bladder and rectum and how, when the mass is removed, the patient will feel much lighter. Meeting the patient in the patient's model of the world would ensure greater rapport, trust, and acceptance of the doctor's findings and suggestions.

The next case shows the opposite representational system mismatch in which a medical social worker is talking with an elderly widowed woman about to be released from the hospital.

MSW: Your doctor feels that you'll be able to leave the hospital soon and return to your apartment.

Patient: I don't know if I can see myself living alone. There'll be no one to look after me.

MSW: I guess you feel a little scared; perhaps you'd be more able to handle going to a nursing home for a while.

Patient: Oh! I can't picture myself in a nursing home. They're all too dull and bleak for me. I don't know if I said this already, I definitely wouldn't go there.

MSW: Do you feel scared living alone?

Patient: I don't know. I just can't see myself as too old to be living alone. Can I stay here a few more weeks until I look better?

MSW: Your doctor doesn't feel you're sick enough to warrant a bed here any more. Perhaps we could arrange for visiting nurses to assist you.

Patient: Can't you see how weak I am? Clearly I'm not ready to go home. I can see the doctor just doesn't care.

MSW: I just don't think you're grasping what I'm saying. He just doesn't feel that. . .

Patient: I see that you don't understand either. It looks like no one cares around here.

Predicates used here should already be obvious. Of course, what the social worker is saying is completely logical and though it may be said in a completely sympathetic and sincere manner (i.e., congruently), the message is not being accepted. All of us have had more than a couple of these similarly frustrating experiences. Again, by taking responsibility for the interchange instead of assigning blame to the elderly woman for being too old or closed-minded to understand, one can meet her in her model of the world and move from there.

Sometimes we meet a friend or patient who we immediately realize speaks the "same language" as we do. It seems very easy to talk to the person and in turn the things the person says seem very sensible and appropriate to us. This compatibility can often be explained by two people having the same primary representational system (rep system). In the same way that you communicate so effectively with people who represent their experiences in a manner similar to yours, by paying attention to rep systems you can approach the same degree of effectiveness with anyone by simply noticing their rep system and modifying your verbal output to be consistent with it. The process of recognizing representational systems must at first be done with some conscious effort. It simply involves noticing the predicates that people use. Though this sounds fairly easy and straightforward, there is often one obstacle. When we listen to someone else, almost all of us are accustomed to hearing only the content of what is being said. When someone is telling us about pain in his right leg we are concentrating appropriately on specific facts such as onset, character, duration, and radiation. However, by concentrating on the content alone, it is difficult to pick up the form or the type of predicates being used. We are not, of course, suggesting that you begin to ignore content. What does work is to set aside a certain specific practice period to listen to just the form of people's language. All of you will have your own particular times when you find this most safe to do. Usually it will be during those times of the day when the content of the conversation you are having is not strictly goal directed, such as when you are setting up some procedure, or while you're making a patient's bed, or during your nonprofessional hours, when talking to a friend or listening to people talking to each other. The important thing is to do it systematically. Set aside a specific amount of time—even if it's only two minutes at a time— when you will pay attention only to form. Even two minutes every other day will be much more useful than just noticing once in a while the key words that people say. After consciously attending to predicates in this manner for awhile, the concentrated effort of doing this will drop out, and it will become second nature to quickly notice a person's major rep system.

REP SYSTEMS AND PACING

With this added tool of knowing in what mode another person organizes his or her experience or reality, the art of pacing can become much more exact and powerful. Not only can the content and nonverbal behavior be mirrored now, but even the very framework in which the person holds all of this. The rewards of attending to and utilizing representational systems should be starting to become obvious to you. When you actually begin to listen to and experience the existence of rep systems in others, you will become aware of the great potential this tool offers in affecting the desired outcomes of any intended communication.

And what about the eye movement patterns, as your eyes defocus momentarily and visualize the movements we were talking about? Remember that listening to predicates will tell you the most favored rep system of a person. Eye movements will simply tell you in what mode a person is experiencing at that moment. This information can have many uses; for our purposes we will discuss some that could be applicable to health professionals. Further uses can be found in the work by Bandler and Grinder.

One very practical use of eye movement patterns is in helping us become aware of when to offer specific bits of information. In any conversation, people usually need time to assimilate within themselves things that have just been said to them. It is precisely when they are in this state that they will miss what you are continuing to offer them. If you systematically begin to notice when people are talking to themselves, or comparing what you have just said with what they have heard previously from others, you can adjust your own output appropriately. Specifically, when most people notice that someone seems to be "somewhere else," they'll talk louder or faster. A workable alternative is to simply pause for as much time as the person needs. Obviously, we don't mean stopping in the middle of a sentence, since that would distract them. Paying attention to people in this manner while offering information and suggestions can ensure that they will at least receive everything that you offer.

Another use of noticing these patterns is in helping patients to verbalize what's on their minds. Often, for example, we are aware that patients seem to be bothered by something, yet when we ask, they don't seem to know what it is. Sometimes people don't want to share it, but frequently they are just not fully conscious of what it is that's troubling them. Instead of asking what they're thinking about, ask them what they're seeing, feeling, or hearing or saying to themselves at that moment, depending on where their eyes are. Asking a patient a question like, "What are you seeing right now, George?" can be so relevant to his experience at that moment that he can easily bring it to the surface and share it. In this case George might have said, "I just saw a picture of the surgeon walking down the hall towards us after my father's surgery." If you had asked what he was thinking he might have said, "Nothing," since in lay terms he was not actually thinking of anything. Similarly, asking what that feeling is, after noticing someone look down and to the right, would be a much more effective route to a person's inner state than just saying something like, "What's wrong?"

Another example was demonstrated by a radiology therapist in Baltimore. As he was about to start a procedure on a patient who was obviously nervous, he saw the patient stop and move her eyes up and to the right. Instead of asking her what she was thinking about, which would have given her time to censor her answers, the therapist asked, "What are you seeing now?" The patient immediately responded that she was seeing herself in the future being sick from the effects of the radiation. The therapist was then easily able to allay her fears with some information that the patient needed. This particular patient was trying to appear strong and unscared. If the therapist had not broken the cycle by asking the question in such a way that the answer wasn't censored, the chances are good that the data about the fear would have been very difficult or impossible to obtain.

Finally, let's return to the previous example involving the nurse who walked into a patient's room with an injection. Recall that the patient's eyes were up and to the left, probably eidetically visualizing a previous scene of himself getting an injection. As we said, eidetic imagery is accompanied by the same feelings that were present in the original situation. Therefore, one strategy might be to assist the patient in becoming unstuck, or less attached to, those feelings of fear. One could do this by eliciting a similar image, but this time with the patient seeing himself in the picture, instead of experiencing being in the picture. This would be analogous to seeing yourself riding the roller coaster, instead of actually experiencing being on the roller coaster and seeing the tracks in front of you. The constructed image would not as strongly elicit the original feelings. Thus, utilizing the sensory experience that the nurse uses to notice that the patient is eidetically visualizing, the nurse might say something like, "I wonder if you're visualizing a previous time when you got an injection; I bet it really hurt. As you notice the doctor or nurse with the needle, and the room you were in, I wonder if you could step outside your body in the picture for a moment so that you can see the whole scene, including yourself sitting or lying there." The result would be a constructed image, having the effect of removing the patient and much of his fear from the past episode. This alone could make the present situation much more palatable. In a following chapter we will talk about the strategy of anchoring and demonstrate how that could be added in a situation like this for even more powerful behavioral results.

Some of the material in this or other chapters may look, feel, or sound as if, in order to use it properly, it would take a lot of studying and concentration. However, we think that the type of study and concentration presented here is not at all like the kind with which you are usually confronted. The effort required to learn these techniques does not involve studying or memorizing written material. It simply demands your attending to sensory experience— going out and starting to consistently notice the form of people's communication patterns, including the body movements that accompany them. Another thing we hope to generate in your behavior is a willingness to try new ways of communicating to people and noticing which ways are successful and which are not. We believe that this type of concentrated effort can be a refreshing and rewarding addition to your present studies, whatever your current level of preparation.

In summary, we each possess different maps on which we represent our experience of reality. There are several ways in which we can represent this reality to ourselves and others. Some of us do this kinesthetically, feeling the world as we go along, attempting to get a good grasp of things. Others primarily see things a certain way, trying to get a clear picture of our situations. Still others mainly listen, attempting to achieve harmony. To stress again, each of us uses all three of the systems; usually, however, one of these is favored— what we are calling a person's primary representational system. Simply listening to the choice of words that people use will reveal their favorite rep system. This is most easily accomplished by first learning to tune out the content of what people are saying and only listen to the form, when it is safe to do so in a given conversation. Recognizing eye patterns can also be an extremely useful tool. While they do not follow the same pattern with everyone, they are always consistent for each person. Therefore noticing in the first thirty seconds or so what an individual's particular pattern is will assist you in knowing how that person organizes his or her thoughts, as well as telling you what system he or she is experiencing in at any particular moment. The uses of this knowledge are limited only by your imagination and willingness to be aware of all the information that people are offering you moment by moment in your interactions with them.

The matching and use of the person's major representational system are particularly effective if incorporated into the techniques of direct communication, indirect communication, and metaphorical communication to be discussed later in this text.

EXERCISES

1. Break up into small groups. Let one person ask questions of a subject that will access visual, auditory, and kinesthetic experiences. Ask five specific questions for each representational system while group members observe the eye movements of the subject and the predicates used in answering the questions.
2. Discuss your preferred representational system of experiencing and those of others you know. How is this expressed or portrayed by interests, vocation, hobbies, or attitudes? As a clinician, how would this information be useful to you?

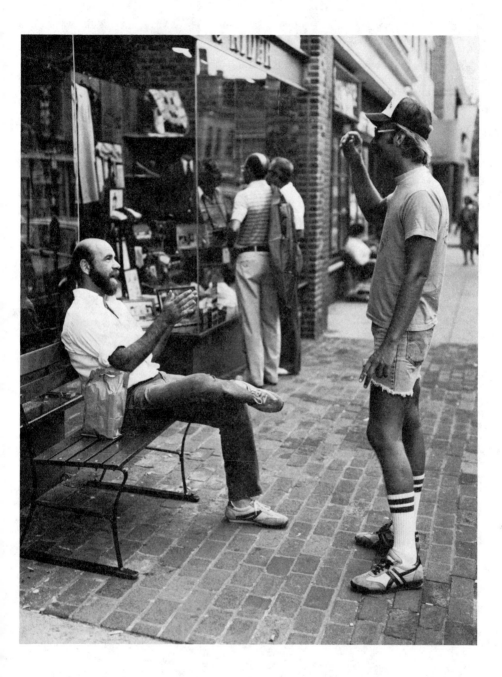

Direct Forms of **4** Communication

In high school many of you probably read the tale about an old sailor who after a long voyage returns home and attends the wedding of his kin. This man desired to become the center of attention at the wedding party and yet, being an effective communicator, he knew he wouldn't hold the interest of the guests by talking in detail about the worlds of navigation or about the structure or even all the specifics of the places he visited. So instead, he begins poetically; "There was a ship quote he," and as he continues

> *He holds them with his glittering eye*
> *The wedding guest stood still,*
> *And listens like a three years' child:*
> *The Mariner hath his will.*

SAMUEL TAYLOR COLERIDGE, *The Rime of the Ancient Mariner*

You already know that *what* you say is only part of the message; however, sometimes (especially when under pressure) you forget that. *How* you say it (i.e., the tones you use, the modulations of your voice, the pauses, the accompanying nonverbal cues) and when you say it are sometimes even more important. For example, the parents who herd their children together, lock the doors, pull down the shades, get close, and whisper, "It's always okay to talk about sex," are not getting their message across—or maybe they are!

Before exploring the aspects of direct and indirect communication, it would no doubt be useful to first review some of the current thinking concerning the way in which we assimilate language. Research over the last few decades suggests that each of the two hemispheres of the brain functions very differently in understanding language. Experiments have been conducted on persons who have had severe damage to one hemisphere and have only the opposite hemisphere intact. Other observations have been carried out on patients who have had commissurotomies. This disconnection of the two halves of the brain by means of surgical severance of the corpus callosum is sometimes done in patients who experience medically uncontrollable seizures. By being able to communicate with one side of the brain at a time, some consistent patterns have been found in the differences between the two hemispheres.

43

The left cerebral hemisphere understands conceptual information. This sentence and the previous few are examples of this. The type of language expressed is objective, logical, analytic, and rational. This is the language of science and reason, explanation, and interpretation. It is also the form of communication that we usually use with patients.

What then remains for the right side of the brain to handle? It is difficult to describe because to do so involves using the left-sided type of language mentioned above. It is described by some as the language of metaphor, analogy, imagery, or symbols. As opposed to the language of analytical dissection, it represents synthesis and tonality. It organizes our experience in a way that transcends words. In this book we will explore methods of communication with each of these hemispheres.

This chapter is mostly a review of things that you have already learned. We will try not to bore you by going over in any detail, or even mention at all in some cases, some of the things that if you haven't learned already you should know from common sense. For example, we will assume that you all know how to listen empathically, creating a generally permissive and accepting atmosphere; this is often important. What we will go over are some of the things associated with direct forms of communication that we consider absolutely critical as base-line skills. Once these direct skills are developed, one can become even more sophisticated by using some of the more creative indirect techniques that we will mention in some detail in Chapter 6.

OBSERVATION

The most important basic tool is the ability to really observe what is happening when interacting with a patient. To be able to look and hear and feel is probably the most important skill any professional communicator can have. A health professional who is a good communicator (which is the only way to be a good health professional) never really has to ask the patient "How are you?" because noticing his or her complexion, skin color, posturing, and movement should reveal the answer to that question before the patient even opens his or her mouth. Putting together verbal and nonverbal cues is a very important part of observation. For example, if a dermatologist who is treating a patient with a skin disorder notices that the patient says, "Oh, my boss has been getting under my skin lately," that dermatologist will know that unless there is some way to help the patient deal with what's going on in his life, all the medicated cream in the world is not going to cure the skin disorder. The patient who comes in slumped over at the shoulders, harried, and depressed with the symptom of back problems, may be helped as much by a simple statement like, "It really is a burden carrying around all that weight on your shoulders— maybe your back will be better when you find some way to relieve some of the load," as they would by twenty hours of physical therapy. The health professional does not need to be a psychiatrist, a psychologist, or a social worker to understand that psychological problems are part of what's going on with the patient, either as part of the etiology or certainly as part of the learned way of being in the world after the illness. One doesn't have to refer the patient to these professionals in order to do some simple psychological treatment as part of the total health care package. (Those of you who still believe in the mind-body split should go directly to jail and do not collect $200.)

Observing people also means observing the representational systems that they use for understanding their world and the strategies they use for making decisions.

CONGRUENCE

The most important issue in direct communication is an emphasis on the congruence of the given message. In the example that we gave previously in this chapter about the parents talking about sex to their children, clearly the problem was the incongruence between their behavior and their words. Equally true, if the health professional is tense, it's very hard to help a patient relax, no matter how sophisticated the techniques he or she may use. If the health professional is genuinely afraid or not interested in people, it is difficult to expect a patient not to be afraid of the health professional or to be comfortable or interested in the situation. A secondary title for this chapter could be "Treating People, Not Patients." One of the important problems often confronting health professionals is their own discomfort with people. It's part of folklore that health professionals often enter their field as a way of doing some personal work for themselves as well as their patients. There is nothing at all wrong with this motive, and in fact, it has probably been one of the prime psychic movers for some of our greatest innovators. The problem is that if somewhere along the line you don't deal with your own plumbing, it's going to be very difficult for you to help anybody else unclog his sink. Oftentimes, especially in moments of crisis (or when we're very harried), it's very difficult to remember that our own attitudes, movements, and responses are some of the most important messages the patients get.

As we write this, we're reminded of the time when two of the authors and one of their children were at an amusement park. We entered a ride that we thought we had some control over in terms of how it moved. When it started, the ride began spinning around in circles quickly and out of our control. One of us said to his seven-year-old daughter at the top of his voice and with a scowled-up face, "Now just relax, just relax!" Even in the midst of the ride, the other author laughed and pointed out, "How do you expect her to relax while you're tense and screaming at her?" It was obvious that the main message that the father was getting across was not one of relaxation, but was in fact a counterproductive message about tension.

LABELS

A rose by any other name may still be a rose—but a person whose name is not used in a way that is comfortable is not a comfortable person. People respond differently to different ways that their name is used. It is very important for a health professional to pace the person's understanding of a name and not to use a "professionally correct" method that might have been learned at the university. Some patients like to be called Mr. Smith, or Dr. Jones, or Reverend Brown; others prefer to be called Linda, or Charlie, or Laurie. It is very easy for a health professional to figure out what to call the person. When you first meet, as you are engaging in the initial greeting (often accompanied by a handshake), it's very easy to say, "Do you prefer to be called Larry or Mr. Clyde?" That question does two things. First, it gets you some information about which way the patient prefers to be called; you can then use that information to communicate in a way that's comfortable for the patient. Second, it conveys to patients that you care about what they want and that you're willing to listen to them—a very important therapeutic message.

One of the authors was having a squamous cell carcinoma removed from his leg and was using trance for an anesthetic. He was fully awake and alert during the procedure. The surgeon, who was not used to awake patients, wanted to make sure everything was okay and said, "How do you feel, son?" The negative feelings of this patient were not just because of the degrading use of "son," but rather because of the knowledge that here was a man cutting open his leg who didn't even know his name.

The three of us usually introduce ourselves to patients as Mark King, Larry Novik, or Charlie Citrenbaum. The patient is then free to call us what they want. The great majority of our patients call us doctor—Doctor King, Doctor Novik, or Doctor Citrenbaum—because they feel more comfortable having a professional relationship with someone called doctor. That of course is fine. However, those people who feel more comfortable with informality and call us Mark, Larry, or Charlie can also have their needs met. We are comfortable enough in our roles that we know we will be the doctor no matter what they call us. None of the procedures will be hindered by any informality.

At the same time that we introduce ourselves and meet the patients, we also find out a little about them: what kind of job they have, who is in their family, what their hobbies are, and so on. Usually, we jot a little bit of this information down on a card or on the patient's chart and glance at it right before their next visit. When they return, we greet them with a question such as, "How's your golf game been going lately?" or "How's that big family of yours?" or "This is your busy season right before tax time, huh?" Again, with minimal effort, we are able to communicate with the patient because we remember something about him or her. (This may be an illusion because we really have to read it from the chart, but it still makes the patient feel good, and therefore, it's a functional illusion.) An important point that needs to be stressed here is that it takes almost no time or effort. Asking people what they like to be called can be done at the initial greeting as they walk in to sit down or as you're initially shaking their hand in the hospital bed. It doesn't take any extra time. Many people have the notion that if you allow patients to talk about themselves or become informal, then somehow it's going to take a lot of extra time, which you can't afford. Others fear this type of relationship creates a buddy-buddy system that's not conducive to a professional working relationship. The only thing that's not conducive to a professional working relationship is an insistence that there's only one correct professional way to do things and that the one way suits all people best.

HIDDEN AGENDAS

Patients often bring hidden agendas to their interactions with health professionals; that is, they talk about one thing or come in with one presenting problem, whereas it's often another thing that worries them or that they would like help in dealing with. They also often come in with a set of expectations that the health professional needs to match if the patients are to be paced effectively. Therefore, we suggest that you find out early on (1) what the patient expects, (2) what they want, and (3) what they're afraid of. These three questions are critical in terms of intake information, and yet one or all of them are often overlooked. How you get this information depends on you and the patient. We can't give you any simple formula, but oftentimes the questions can be straight and directly asked. Other times, the answers may need to be intuited. It's just important for you to remember that what the patient tells you initially is usually not the full story; you have to look for the meaning between the lines and listen to what the patient does not say.

A good illustration of this can be found in patients who come to a doctor for a physical examination. With the exception of those who come in to get required forms filled out, most other patients have a specific reason for why they choose a particular day or week for an appointment. In the authors' experience, they usually do not communicate that specific reason at first. It is only after sometimes repeated questioning that the majority of people admit to a specific problem or fear. Sometimes it is that a close friend just suffered a heart attack or that one of their parents died of cancer at the age they are now approaching. Other times it is because they are feeling depressed and they are wondering if maybe something physical is causing their symptoms. Often it is an attempt to procure information about touchy subjects such as sex.

Another common example is the familiar "pain in the ass" patient who keeps calling the nurses to his or her room every ten minutes. Behind many of these people's behavior lies a powerful fear or helplessness. By getting nurses and aides to come, they get at least some sense of control. When standing in front of a nagging patient, it is immeasurably easier for health professionals to be with them if they can sense the fear, sadness, or helplessness that often is engulfing the patient and to help him or her recognize and begin to deal with it.

SELF-FULFILLING PROPHECIES

One of the best ways to modify behavior is to casually mention to the client what are commonly called self-fulfilling prophecies. Statements can be made about what you believe will or won't happen in a very casual, matter-of-fact way. For example, if you're a health professional working with another health professional who is the patient, you can casually make the statement, "I know professional people know a lot about their bodies and therefore their healing process is faster." Or if you're working with parents and you want them to modify their behavior in terms of what they're doing with their children, you could make the statement, "I know that you're good parents and that you always know what to do that's best and therefore you will do so-and-so, I'm sure." It creates the self-fulfilling prophecy that they're good parents, which of course they want to believe anyway, and that therefore they're going to do what you tell them to do. Telling people good things about themselves, if it is at all in pace with how they feel or want to feel, followed by a statement such as, "Because you're like this, I know that you will do so-and-so," almost always produces the desired behavior. The technique is particularly effective when used in conjunction with junko logic, an indirect communication technique to be discussed later in this text.

The whole idea of using casual conversation and matter-of-fact ways of behavior to direct a patient to do things that might ordinarily seem out of his or her ability is a very effective technique. We know a dentist who often tells patients in a very matter-of-fact way to "turn off the saliva now" and is able to produce a dry field to work with very easily. If this dentist had made a big production of this particular direction, chances are the majority of patients would not have been able to do it. Any authority figure (and certainly health professionals represent such an authority to dependent patients) can get almost anybody to do anything if they state it in such a way that it seems normal, natural, expected, and easy to do. It is also important to modify comments that can be negative self-fulfilling prophecies. One well-known example is about the mother who takes her son to the clinical psychologist and says, "Doctor, I don't know why he doesn't feel good about himself. Each morning I tell him 'Shorty, you're as good as anyone else.' "

NEGATIONS

Negations are very ineffective words to use in communication, for two reasons. First, they tempt the consciousness of the person to show its independence by not following the directions. Second, there is evidence to demonstrate that the unconscious or right side of the brain does not pick up negation, which would then make the message contradictory to each hemisphere. The following are some obvious examples of this.

As gamblers, the authors are all willing to bet that right now not one of you could put your thumb lightly over the edge of the left side of this book and not think of the word elephant. When you say to a person, "this won't hurt much," you're essentially telling them it's going to hurt. The word "much" means different things to different people, and while it's quite debatable and variable, there is no doubt that the part of the message that they're picking up is "this is going to hurt."

RELABELING

A common technique that helps you avoid negation is the process of relabeling. Since particular words have specific good feelings that are elicited when they are spoken, it is helpful to use these in lieu of phrases with negation. If your interest is to let the patient know that something is going to be felt, but that it won't be too bad, you can relabel hurt to a tickle or pressure sensation. If you tell them they're going to feel some pressure and that it may tickle a little — but don't laugh too hard, you have redefined the feeling and set up a self-fulfilling prophecy of its not hurting. Many doctors before examining children's ears will say something like, "Now I want you to promise me that you're not going to laugh too much because this might really tickle!" Note that the negation here obviously causes laughing before the ears are even touched.

We don't want health professionals to lose their credibility and we're not suggesting you do this on procedures you know to be extremely painful. However, it's very common to make statements like, "this won't hurt much," about procedures that in fact don't hurt certain people at all and in others result only in minor pressure or irritation at most. In addition to avoiding using negations in general, it's best to leave out any kind of word that implies something difficult or painful. It's generally not a good practice to tell people that they'll need to work hard with you during this procedure, or in the physical therapy, and so on. Hard work carries a negative connotation for most people. Occasionally it may be useful to give a person a pep talk using this term, and for some people who are in fact very hard workers it may set a good pace, but for most it's rather a negative concept.

One of us was recently sitting in the dentist's office going through the laborious task of having his teeth cleaned, but doing so in a totally relaxed manner, drifting off into dreamland and enjoying himself. He was suddenly rudely interrupted by the dental hygienist, who said, "I want you to open your mouth very wide." Both the words and the tone used by the hygienist implied something that was a lot of hard work to a person who was sitting there quite relaxed and enjoying himself. It would have been more helpful for the hygienist to have said to the person, "Since you're sitting there so relaxed, I'd like you to relax your jaw even more so that your mouth can open even wider." That is an excellent pace since the hygienist is first seeing what the person is already doing, recognizing it and repeating it back, and then leading the person to a new behavior that will result in the intensification of the original behavior.

When using direct oral communication it's very important to be careful of what contract words you make with client. For example, we never ask someone to "try" something and we never say "if," because both "if" and "try" are examples of contract words that imply the possibility, and sometimes even the probability, of failure. Trying to stop smoking doesn't help your lungs, stopping smoking does. "If you take" your medicine doesn't get anybody better, "taking" your medicine is what matters. As opposed to "if" and "try," "when" is a good word to use because it implies that it's going to happen—the only debatable point is whether it's going to happen now or a little while from now.

Again, this particular part relates to the illusion of choice method that will be elaborated in Chapter 6.

CHANGING TENSE

Another way to simply effect change when it's appropriate is to change the tense of what you or the patient is saying. If you've just directed a patient to stop smoking and you want to discuss it, don't discuss what happens with smoking in the present tense. Instead, ask the patient what were the reasons he or she used to smoke. In a well-known case of his, Milton Erickson was working in psychotherapy with a client to help her get unstuck from an emotion she was carrying around from an earlier traumatic experience. He had her relive that experience in her fantasy. As she was getting excited, he emotionally said, "That hurts terribly—didn't it?" The change of tense in the middle of the sentence helped her to both consciously and unconsciously put the pain in the perspective of the past.

One of the authors saw an agoraphobic who had temporarily freed herself just enough from her disorder to venture to his office. She never in her life had driven further away from home than his office, which was only about 20 minutes away. She had also never driven the car alone. Always accompanying her to the office was her 24-year-old son, who had just been released from the Marine Corps, and usually the son's fiancée. On one occasion the author was late for a scheduled appointment. He apologized, but the woman said, "Well, I have nothing to do anyway. I just stay around the house all day." The author said "Yes, but I'm also keeping your son waiting." The woman just took a deep sigh and said, "Oh, I'd like to go someplace without him." Using the technique of anchoring, which will be described in Chapter 8, the author helped her on with her coat and walked her downstairs past her son and into the car, touching her right shoulder the whole time. He directed her to go to a hill (because she really liked hills and used them a lot in her fantasy work) in a park about two miles from the office. As the author walked back to his office, the son asked, "Where's my mother?" and the author said, "She's doing a task, she'll be back soon." The son and fiancée ran outside to discover the car was gone and then proceeded to pace back and forth outside for about 15 minutes. The author watched this with some amusement and when the pacing increased, he decided that he needed to go down and do some family intervention, lest he become the victim of what seemed like an imminent assault. Just as he got downstairs, the mother came back, pulled up in the car, and ran up the steps all excited. The author greeted the mother and they walked together past the son and fiancée. As they passed, the son said to the author, "You don't understand, my mother just doesn't drive by herself," whereupon the author turned to him and said, "You're right, she didn't, did she?"

ELICITING QUESTIONS

Another very effective direct communication technique that helps you get the client's attention is to set up a situation in which the client asks for information before you first offer it. As an example, if you would like to explain to a patient the relationship between tension and pain as a motivation to help him or her relax before doing a procedure, you may say to a co-worker who is there with you, "Mary Jane's coming in next, isn't she?" After receiving an affirmative reply from the co-worker, you could say, "Good, because I really want to use the dental probe and fist example to help demonstrate to her the value of relaxation. I know she'll enjoy it." Chances are your patient will be curious so that he or she will either outrightly ask you what you're talking about or at least show some signs of curiosity. You could then explain to your patient exactly what you wanted to do.

PARALLEL EXAMPLES

Another technique for effective communication is utilizing parallel examples. Although we probably all already make use of these, examples need to be mentioned so that we can have conscious appreciation of them and use them more often when appropriate. Examples from childhood are particularly potent. These are different from metaphors, which will be discussed in a separate chapter, in that parallel examples are quite obvious and direct and meant for the conscious attention of the person. A hospitalized patient is about to have a transfusion and is giving the nurse a difficult time. He says that he had one of these when he was younger and he recalls how incredibly painful it was and how sore his arm was for weeks afterward. The nurse reminds him about how when he used to play on a hill behind his house, it probably seemed so gigantic and powerful; yet now that he's grown up, when he goes back and looks at it, it seems so small that he wonders how he could have even possibly found it exciting. The nurse reminds him how we all exaggerate things, both positive and negative, from our childhood memories. The nurse could then turn this into a self-fulfilling prophecy by telling him that he's going to be surprised by how painless this procedure is going to be.

A group of parallel examples that were made famous by Milton Erickson are called early learning sets. These are things that the three authors use quite frequently in their work with patients. Oftentimes when a health professional is working with a patient, the patient feels that the task at hand is insurmountable. It's important to remind patients of the whole history they have in growing up—of doing things that seemed very difficult, even impossible at the time, and yet today those same things are so commonplace and ordinary that they can't even remember when they were difficult. You can talk about learning to walk and have them just imagine how they got up and then fell back down . . . and they got up and they fell back down again—but eventually learned to stand on their own two feet and walk . . . and now it's so ordinary and everyday for them to do that; even though it's not even two o'clock, they've probably already taken a thousand steps today. . . . We often reminisce about learning the alphabet and how difficult it seemed to learn the difference between an "M" and an "N," an "O" and a "Q," and to learn one's name and numbers . . . and just as you get that down how they changed from printing to script and you had to start all over again. It's so easy for them to read and write, yet they can't even tell us the process by which they do it—it's already unconscious and automatic. To remind people that they have the resources, the ability, and the history of facing seemingly impossible tasks helps them get in touch with those resources and use that personal power as needed in the present.

DIRECTIVES

As we mentioned in Chapter 1, it is often a good idea to give patients directives; that is, tasks to carry out when they're not with you. This may not be necessary for a physical therapist in the middle of an intense case who sees the client every day, but for a social worker who may see a family only occasionally or a physician dealing with someone having a problem whom they see only once every two or three weeks, it allows the patients to take an active part in their own treatment during the time between sessions with you and to understand that treatment is also taking place between sessions. For example, we think it is very important to give people who have health problems directives about exercising. By this we mean not just the general notion that it's good to exercise, but even some specific exercises. At home every day the patients will then know that they are doing something actively positive to facilitate their own treatment. Another factor is that you are better able to do your work when the client comes to you after spending time at home following your directives. A significant problem for professionals doing psychological work is that they see patients only once a week. By not receiving directives, the patients get the message that basically the work they'll do for personal growth will be only during this one hour a week and is in a way detached from the rest of their life. We have given patients books that we thought might be good for them to read, and we've told them specific places to read the books. We've often directed them to make an hour's trip to a certain park and climb on certain rocks out by the waterfalls to read a particular book. Once a client goes to all that trouble to read the book, they'll expend more energy toward understanding what it is about than if they just casually sat down at home and read parts of it at their convenience.

The whole idea of directives is beautifully illustrated by the expanding field of nutrition. While many aspects of this science have been medically proven, there are still many claims that are purely theoretical, but espoused enthusiastically by some of its followers. The one thing that is plainly true, however, is that many if not most people *do* feel a positive and therapeutic effect when switching to one of these diet regimens. Whether this is a placebo effect or not is largely open to conjecture. Examples of this are sugar and food additive elimination diets in hyperactive children and megavitamin therapy in the treatment of many other disorders.

One indisputable fact is that when people actually change their diet they are taking an active, continuing role in their own healing process. They are also taking some responsibility for their own bodies instead of leaving their problems to the health professional to work on for several minutes every week or two. If in fact we discover in the future that many of these dietary approaches do actually make a difference biochemically, it will still, we believe, not have as powerful an effect as the self-responsibility denominator we have talked about.

IDENTIFICATION WITH ANOTHER

Another exotic and somewhat tricky technique that you may want to experiment with, and one that we ourselves are just beginning to incorporate into our work, is having the patient take on the identity, or at least some characteristics, of other people who are able to do things that they are not. A social worker friend of ours was called into the hospital to deal with a patient management problem. This patient had a very low self-esteem. She was to undergo a serious procedure and the physicians had some concern about her ability to survive the operation. The social worker saw her the night before and tried to make some kind of contact through traditional ways and was totally unsuccessful, going home frustrated (as we all have at times). She thought about it that night and she promptly marched herself in the hospital at 5:30 A.M. the next morning. She walked to the startled woman's bed and said, "You're not worth a hill of beans; your body is falling apart, your mind is falling apart, you cause trouble for everyone here, and I know you can't make it through this operation" (a perfect pace because this is exactly what the woman felt). "But you know that I could make it through this operation, so why don't you just become me for the next three hours?" She then turned and walked out the door. She was called that afternoon by the hospital staff asking what the hell she did because the patient sailed through the procedure and was now pleasant as could be. You can often ask patients who are struggling with particular issues to imagine people whom they know either in reality or from fiction, characters from books or television, for example, and to think about how these people, whom they admire and whom they believe could deal with what they are struggling with, might go about dealing with this issue. This often allows them to come up with some very creative problem-solving techniques.

SECONDARY GAINS AND REFRAMING

It is critical that every health professional remember that almost all long-term discomfort and disability is accompanied by some positive gains. Treating the disorder also requires dealing with these secondary gains of the patient. For example, the person who is disabled and has been out of work for a year, while genuinely wanting to get better, still has to recognize that there is something positive about not having to go to work, about not being responsible within the family, and about being nurtured in a way that children often are by their parents. This is not to blame the person for the disorder or accuse the person of malingering; however, it is important for health professionals to recognize that for almost all long-term disorders at least a few changes take place within the social structure of that patient's life that are positive, even if they have a hard time consciously recognizing these facts.

Have you ever wondered at the amazing amount of secondary gain behind the usual type of fainting? When someone is in a frightening and threatening situation, a vasovagal reaction may occur in which the blood vessels suddenly dilate, thereby pooling blood in the lower extremities. Blood flow to the brain is consequently diminished and the person thus experiences a loss of consciousness. The secondary gain is obvious—an immediate escape from the threat involved. You will note that people rarely faint in the middle of a busy street or when their child is badly injured (at least until the nurse or doctor arrives). We're not saying that a person makes a conscious choice to have this attack, but only that there is definitely an unconscious appreciation of the secondary gains that ensue.

Another wonderful example of secondary gains occurs with migraine headache sufferers. In its classic description, the pain of a migraine can be alleviated only by lying still in a quiet, dark room for 12 to 24 hours. What a deal! No work, no clothes to pick up at the cleaners, no straightening up around the apartment, and no guilt about not going to work and leaving everyone to cover (how can you go to work if you've got the worst headache in the world!). How many of you get a 12 to 24 hour break like that once or twice a month? Again, we're not accusing people of consciously choosing these headaches nor are we belittling the severity of these excruciating episodes. We also realize that people would truly give anything to rid themselves of these headaches. Before they will go away permanently, however, the secondary gains must be appreciated by the patient.

This phenomenon is utilized by the authors in treatment of migraine patients. After the secondary gains are explored, patients are told that they need to make time in their schedules for completely free evenings at least several times a week. When it was shown that the patients were actually observing this free time every few days with regularity, the incidence of headaches dropped precipitously.

One of the best ways that we know of to deal with secondary gains is a technique that Bandler and Grinder call reframing. Bandler and Grinder often use this technique in trance at an unconscious level, but we have found it extremely effective at a conscious level in just straight talking to the person.

The technique of reframing essentially affirms to the person that there is some payoff or benefit from the symptom and that it's okay to keep these payoffs, but that there may be better ways that they could keep the benefits and yet not have to have some of the dysfunction. You can work with the person to help them come up with some of the possible payoffs for their behavior and to come up with alternatives that could get them the same payoffs without the dysfunction. You could then encourage them to go out and try them and see which ones seem to work and how they affect the disorder.

As an example, every health professional knows that smoking is an unhealthy dysfunctional behavior. (Unfortunately 30 to 40 per cent of you reading this book are probably smokers; some of you are probably smoking as you are reading this.) When you are working with a smoker, instead of simply ordering them to stop (because if there were no secondary gains involved, many would be able to just summon up the will power, throw the cigarettes in the trash can, and walk away), you can patiently talk about the idea of secondary gains and in fact engage them in this process we call reframing.

To illustrate, here is a discussion that took place between a clinical social worker and a patient who came for help to stop smoking. The patient, a 50-year-old business executive, has beginning signs of emphysema and has been told by his physician that he must stop smoking. However, he has been futilely trying to stop for weeks.

Social worker:	Do you believe that in some way smoking has had payoffs or benefits for you?
Patient:	No way! It's a disgusting, unhealthy habit, but I just can't stop.
Social worker:	Well, just for the sake of discussion, would you be willing to assume for a few minutes that, in some way, smoking has payoffs for you?
Patient:	Okay, I can assume that.
Social worker:	Good, now we have to communicate and work with that part of you that's been responsible for your smoking. I know that you're going to stop smoking only when that part of you is satisfied to do so. (This communication tends to defuse and parcel out some of the normal resistance to change a patient would often experience.) What I'd like to ask you to do is to close your eyes and relax and take a few moments and in some way experience that part of you that's been responsible for your smoking—it may be something you'll see or something you'll hear or think in your mind or maybe something you'll feel.
Patient:	(After having his eyes closed about 30 seconds, he surprisingly reports that he sees the face of his deceased father.)
Social worker:	That's interesting. Did your father smoke cigarettes?
Patient:	As a matter of act, he did. They finally killed him. He died of lung cancer at the age of 56 (teary-eyed). I loved him and always felt guilty that he died so young. I wish we had spent more time together.
Social worker:	I wonder if you're taking care of your guilt by trying to kill yourself with cigarettes?
Patient:	I never thought of that.
Social worker:	Would you be willing to close your eyes again and, in your imagination, have a conversation with your father about your smoking? Ask him if it's all right for you to stop smoking and live a lot longer than he did.
Patient:	(After having eyes closed for a munute.) It's all right. I've also decided to make a yearly contribution to the American Cancer Society.
Social worker:	Good. Now I think you'd better explore whether there have been any other payoffs from your smoking cigarettes. Will you close

Patient:	your eyes again and come up with any other possible payoffs. (Closes his eyes a few moments and then reports a tightness in his chest.)
Social worker:	Does that tightness mean anything to you or remind you of anything?
Patient:	Yes, it's the same tightness I get at the office. When it happens I stop what I'm doing and have a cigarette and relax. I guess another payoff is that having a cigarette is relaxing—it gives me an excuse to take a break.
Social worker:	Do you need an excuse to take a break? I want to suggest to you that at least once every hour when you're working, you stop, take a few deep breaths of air, and relax for at least five to ten minutes.
Patient:	Okay, that sounds great.
Social worker:	Now will you close your eyes again and make sure that part of you that's been responsible for your smoking in the past will be satisfied that you don't smoke, but that instead you'll engage in the new alternative behaviors we've been discussing.
Patient:	(After having his eyes closed a few moments) My father was smiling and my chest was relaxed. Everything is okay.
Social worker:	Great. And I'd like to thank you for the good work you've done here today.

To summarize, here are the suggested basic steps in the reframing process:

1. Get the patient to accept that the dysfunctional pattern of behavior or experience (let's call it X) has had a payoff or payoffs for him or her.

2. Ask the patient to experience in some way that part of himself or herself that's been responsible for X. Express your desire to work with that part of the patient.

3. Ask the patient to identify the payoffs for X.

4. Ask your patient to identify alternative patterns of behavior that can provide the same payoffs but be more functional and healthy.

5. Make sure that the alternative patterns will be satisfactory.

The health professional may often have to help the patient identify payoffs and alternative patterns. All of the above steps do not necessarily need to be applied. And in some cases, the health professional may have to be creative in generating other steps when helping the patient to engage in the reframing process.

This chapter has been a review of some very useful straightforward techniques for interacting effectively with patients. These ideas are not meant to be glanced over just once. We urge you to review the topics and see which ones could be useful to you. Becoming familiar with these techniques greatly increases the likelihood that you will find yourself utilizing them in the very near future.

We end this chapter with a paper by a man we know to be an outstanding communicator as a health professional. The author is a pediatrician on the staff of Children's Hospital in Pittsburgh, Pennsylvania. While only a very small percentage of people reading this book will be pediatricians, the principles in the paper are generalizable to any of your fields. It is a good demonstration of taking the principles that we have previously discussed and showing how they can be applied to a specific area. We are sure your own creative skills will allow you to do the same in your own area of interest. We ask you to pay special attention to the way the author paces the parents (especially their fears) and listens closely to understand what the parents are really meaning by what they say, and how he effectively communicates with them.

ESTABLISHING EFFECTIVE PARENT/PATIENT COMMUNICATION

WILLIAM I. COHEN, M.D.
Clinical Assistant Professor of Pediatrics
University of Pittsburgh
School of Medicine
Pittsburgh, Pennsylvania

A fundamental goal of primary care pediatrics is the promotion of the optimum development and functioning of the individual child—leading to an adult who is able to productively function to his or her maximum potential. Realization of this goal entails an awareness that contemporary health care goes far beyond simply "taking care" of patients during acute illness. It requires a sound knowledge of the fundamental elements of child development and behavior, their normal progression over time, and the ways in which they can be impacted upon by acute, as well as chronic changes in the child's internal or external environment. To effectively mobilize this knowledge for the benefit of his patients, the primary care pediatrician must acknowledge that he is a *facilitator* and *translator* for the true "care givers"—the parents or other responsible individuals. They play the primary role of day-to-day observation and management of the physical, developmental, and emotional health of the child. The pediatrician is clearly dependent upon them to provide him with the data base upon which he can form his hypotheses and to efficaciously carry out his management plans. Appropriate diagnostic formulation and intervention demands understanding the child and parents on their own terms in a nonjudgmental fashion. Clearly, this requires good rapport and open lines of communication between the pediatrician and care givers. Therefore, in order for the pediatrician to be of greater service to parents and therefore the child, it is imperative that this relationship be established from early on and its nature characterized, including its limitations from both parental and physician's perspectives.

In order for the pediatrician to effectively counsel and advise his patients (including the parents of his patients), he must understand the physical, social, and emotional milieu of the family and also have continuous feedback from the child and parent as he forms his hypotheses and therapeutic plans. To maximize the validity of his decision making, he must have a strong data base, which in the case of well child care and issues of development and behavior is generated in large part from history obtained from the parents. Many of the presenting behavioral and developmental dysfunctions may not be readily visible to the physician during the short period of the office evaluation during which a multitude of factors can interfere with reliable assessment of a child's current functional status. A carefully taken history can serve several purposes in this regard: it can provide a precise description of a developmental and behavioral parameter *over time* (simultaneous sampling of a parameter in several environments enhancing validity); it can serve to focus the physician's hands-on assessment to be more efficient; and importantly, it gives insights into the parents' perceptions of the problem that may significantly impact on their ability to carry out a therapeutic plan. Therefore, it is obvious that the physician must cultivate within his patients a sense of ease about communicating their concerns to him and, in turn, responding openly to his inquiries.

Toward this end, there are several general guidelines that the physician can follow in his interactions with his patients. At a most basic level, every interview should begin with an open-ended question regarding the patient's or parents' concerns about the child at this moment in time (e.g., "What brought you here today?" for acute situations and, "What concerns do you have?" for child maintenance situations). Open-ended questioning will frequently give more pertinent information than running through a checklist of questions designed to be comprehensive but not specific. The concerns raised should be addressed point by point during the evaluation to specifically answer each question. Frequently, concerns may seem to be of trivial nature—these should not be brushed aside with sayings like "there's no problem" or "that's okay." Such nonchalant responses may miss important underlying fears and communicate disinterest. It is important to realize that while the contact may only be a brief one in a long day for the physician, it may very well be the single most important event for the family in several months. No concern can be considered too trivial. A casual response to a real concern may be the main message taken away. It is the obligation of the pediatrician to be sensitive to the verbal and nonverbal communication of the parents in an attempt to assess their level of concern about any particular issue. When the parent returns to a question somewhat later on in the interview or seems dissatisfied either verbally or with a frown, the pediatrician must then attempt to root out the cause for the concern. Such a question as, "What was it about this that concerned you?" or "What did you think was the problem?" will help disclose the hidden agendas or concerns. Although a particular symptom may seem trivial, it may have deep meaning to the parent because of an episode in the past, experience of a neighbor, etc. By not addressing these concerns directly in a supportive fashion, satisfaction and therefore compliance drop off markedly.

The importance of developing good listening skills cannot be overemphasized. It is necessary to develop the *willingness* to listen to the patient and parent and accept their communications as valid statements of the way they have experienced the world and specifically their medical problems. The pediatrician knows the child or infant better than the parents only for a few hours at the beginning of life. Thereafter, the child's behavior and activities are known best to his primary caretakers. Therefore, any information that they impart to the physician must be respected. That is not to say that it should be accepted without a critical eye. Clearly, stress, fatigue, and misplaced concern can modify parents' ability to report accurately. Nevertheless, the basic facts should be solicited carefully and then addressed point by point. Even if the physician is not concerned about a specific symptom, the fact that the parent is means that this issue must be addressed and the parents reassured. The physician must acknowledge the parents' level of concern and address it directly by explaining the reasons why he is not concerned or by acknowledging that it is an issue that needs to be pursued further. The further investigation of a problem area initially involves follow-up appointments with the primary care physician for monitoring and further definition of the course of a specific problem over time. Diagnostic tests, therapeutic-trial intervention, or referral to another health care provider are second-line responses that should be done in a logical and systematic fashion. In any event, continuing feedback should be sought so that the implications of the condition whether significant or benign are understood by the parents.

The physician must keep in mind that guilt is ever present when a medical condition is discovered in a child and some step should be immediately taken to address the parental guile. In the case of a significant condition that may have long-term effects, care should be taken that the parents have been provided with an accurate explanation of the condition at the time of initial recognition. This should address their perceptions and fears about the problem. Dealing with these issues from the onset greatly enhances the parents' ability to appropriately respond. Such information is best given in the presence of both parents so that misunderstanding does not occur when one parent attempts to transmit this to the other. This information will need to be transmitted again during follow-up visits, each time defining parents' perceptions and directly addressing emerging fears.

Physicians make assumptions about the competence of parents that can be damaging to both members in the dyad. Parents who are health professionals (nurses, physicians, psychologists, and pharmacists, for example) frequently are assumed to have special competence in child rearing on the basis of their exposure in their professional training to issues of child health. In fact, parental responsibility and its resultant feelings and responses transcend educational work or other experiences. No assumptions whatsoever should be made on the part of health professionals as to the parents' understanding of any symptom or disease process. Rather, the assumption can more rightly be made that on the basis of small amounts of incomplete information that the parents have, any one symptom's importance is liable to be magnified and taken out of proportion. (The physician only need think about his own reaction to a symptom in his child and all the possible implications that pertain thereto.) Consequently, it behooves the physician to overstate to the parents that the physician makes no assumptions whatsoever about the parents' level of knowledge or expertise in these matters and consequently, they should not hesitate to ask questions that are concerning them. (Medically sophisticated parents may need to be told that they might have a need to ask more questions, inasmuch as the knowledge that they do have will call to mind many more concerns.) The parents are told that there are no "dumb" questions. In fact, the concept of the dumb question reflects that particular parent's erroneous expectation that they know the answer.

A role of the pediatrician should be one of supporting the parents' ability to make increasing numbers of independent judgments about child care and child health. Therefore, it should be the goal of the pediatrician to encourage and foster the development of good observational skills on the part of the parents. These observations then can be integrated with information previously presented to them so that at any given point, the parent is able to confidently pursue a rational plan for management of any episode. The parent must be able to make some basic judgments as to the severity of an acute illness and how to proceed—whether with watchful waiting, simple home interventions, or consultation with the physician. What decision is made will be based on the objective findings in the child, the parents' ability to see the symptoms without projecting outcome on the basis of past experiences with illness, and the success in managing past episodes of acute illness. Parents frequently call on the pediatrician at these times for advice. Parents who are unsure of their ability to read their child's symptoms, or who have not been educated with respect to what factors to attend to, may present with complaints that the pediatrician, at a casual glance, will find annoying and bothersome. A pediatrician who is not sensitized to parental concerns may get quite annoyed at such calls inasmuch as the child clearly is not severely ill. The physician who asks curtly, "Why are you calling me now for such a minor episode?" fails to pace the parents and appears to be unaware of their behavior as a response to a fear that had been inculcated by parents' friends, previous experiences, or perhaps other physicians. In addressing parent anxiety in these situations, the physician must again move beyond the presenting symptom and directly address parent concerns—"Is there something special you are concerned about?" Once this is accomplished, it is necessary to begin to educate the parents to the salient features that must be observed when a child is ill. By shifting parental focus to the features of the child he concerns himself with, the pediatrician is able to begin the step of re-educating parents and training them to be better observers. Specific instructions on the use of selective treatment modalities for given conditions and instructions on when to contact the physician should there be a change in symptomatology can then be given. This systematic approach greatly enhances parental satisfaction and compliance.

The time spent in listening to, reassuring, and educating parents will reap benefits the next time the child presents with a similar situation. They will feel able to make preliminary assessments and treatment by themselves and feel free to contact the physician if they are uncomfortable with the situation as it progresses. Parents need to be reinforced that the physician is available to help them in their caretaking and that when a question arises about the child's health, behavior, or activity, it is appropriate to ask the physician. It is comforting to the parents to know that they do not have to make these decisions alone, especially since this would then place the burden of guilt on them should there be unfavorable outcome from one of their decisions. By encouraging frequent telephone or other contact early on in the relationship, the pediatrician promotes confidence building in the parents and in the long run liberates physician and parent alike. Some individuals may abuse this privilege either because of lack of maturity, inability to make decisions, or for other idiosyncratic reasons. This should be dealt with on a case-by-case basis through spending more time educating and describing discrepancies between the level of concern and the child's actual health during regular office visits or specially arranged consultations. A high degree of sustained parental anxiety is in itself a symptom and needs to be addressed in a comprehensive and nonjudgmental fashion. This may include further exploration of basic aspects of the parent/child relationship and factors that may be interfering such as other stress events in the lives of the parents.

Frequently, parents will call when a child has either had a symptom for a short period of time or, on the other hand, for a rather extended period of time. The physician's immediate reaction may be "Why did you call so soon?" or "Why did you wait so long?" The accusatory nature of this communication is extremely damaging and puts a tremendous burden of guilt on the parents. It is obvious that they called when they did because they had lost the ability to deal with the symptom with their own resources. Therefore, the appropriate question is not "Why did you call so soon?" but "What is it about this symptom that caused you to be so concerned at this time?" Likewise, when a parent calls after a prolonged duration of a symptom, the appropriate line of inquiry includes a statement such as "Can you tell me what's different now that led you to call?" This line of questioning avoids accusations and more importantly is an approriate attempt to learn from parents the nature of their concerns. Except for situations of an extremely emergent nature, the physician should defer addressing his concerns, which are not identified as problem areas by the parent, until after parent concerns are addressed. Failure to do so can cause a schism in parent/physician communication. Investigation should be minimized in areas of questionable importance to the presenting problem, in order to avoid friction between the individuals, When a physician does identify a significant problem of which the parents are not aware, he must sensitize them to the significance of the problem in terms of its long-range outcome. By identifying the area as one of concern, he may wish to acknowledge that he understands that though the parents may not feel uncomfortable with the present situation and therefore not understand the reason for concern, presenting the logical outcome will serve to refocus the parents on the health hazard (e.g., the night-time bottle and nursing bottle caries). The pediatrician should make the appropriate interventions and recommendations with follow-up directed toward monitoring the parents' understanding of the concerns and their change in behavior. The physician should guard against messages that imply that the parents are incompetent for allowing behaviors to occur that the parents did not know were potentially dysfunctional.

It should be ovious that these guidelines do not pertain to pediatrics alone, but really are skills that should be acquired by anyone in the health care professions inasmuch as they are basic to the ability to understand a health care issue and then intervene appropriately. The physician must listen attentively to parents or patients and try to understand their model of reality as they have experienced it. Then using his own skills and understanding of disease and human interactional processes, he must attempt to appropriately direct the parents' focus as necessary and intervene. He can only be successful when he understands the patient/parents' concerns and begins to address these point by point.

EXERCISES

1. Each of the following phrases or sentences violates a principle or concept of effective communication that has been presented in this chapter. Identify the principle(s) or concept(s) that applies and correct the phrase accordingly.
   a. "Don't think about your upcoming surgery."
   b. "Try to take your medicine on schedule."
   c. "Many people have had difficulty with this procedure. I hope that you won't."
   d. "This medicine shouldn't make you feel too nauseous."
2. Discuss five gains that you or your patients can possibly get in life from being sick.

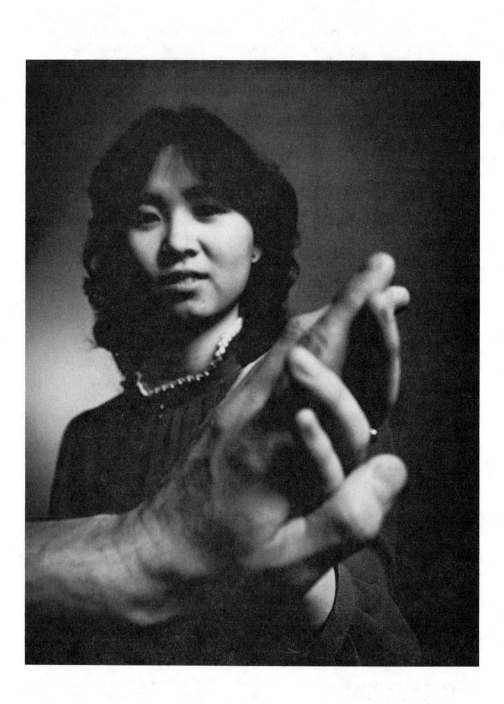

Nonverbal 5 Communication

What people do is often more important than what they say.

Milton Erickson is legendary for the remarkable skill he displayed in his observation and use of nonverbal behavior. In his teaching, seminars, and writings, Erickson constantly stressed the importance of nonverbal cues for effective communication. One of his favorite anecdotes concerned a new patient who upon entering Erickson's office immediately expressed pessimism that Erickson could be helpful. The man went through a long, detailed story listing all the well-known therapists who had failed to help him during the last year. Erickson had never met this young man before, nor had he received any information about him. However, he confidently stated that he could ask the patient one question that would convince him of Erickson's skill and knowledge. The man accepted the challenge, and Erickson asked, "How long have you been a man?" The patient was amazed at Erickson's "mindreading" and was won over. The patient had recently undergone a sex change operation and was experiencing difficulty adjusting. Erickson had noticed the man extended his right arm out from his chest when he lifted a piece of lint from his left shoulder. Erickson knew that only a woman avoiding her breasts would display this movement. The young man had continued to engage in that habitual pattern of behavior after his operation.

Erickson, of course, was not the first to stress the importance and power of nonverbal communication. Many social scientists have described our extreme sensitivity and responsiveness to bodily movement and gestures and how our relationships are regulated and maintained without regard to language and consciousness. In their now classic statement of the double-bind theory of schizophrenia, Bateson and associates (1956) illustrated the stress produced by a verbal parental message ("Come give me a big hug") paired with an incongruent nonverbal message (standing rigid and cold when the hug is given).

The last twenty years have ushered in a great deal of interest and research in nonverbal communication. Productivity was increased by the use of modern devices such as videotape equipment and sophisticated sound filtering ma-

---

Thanks to Robert Henderson, M.S.W., for his contributions to this chapter.

chines, which can preserve the emotional tone of speech but otherwise mask its meaning.

As one example of these studies, Robert Rosenthal and colleagues (1973) supported the power of nonverbal cues through the use of a measure they developed called the PONS test, which gauged sensitivity to nonverbal communication. They produced 200 film segments of an actress nonverbally expressing various emotions in certain contexts. The experimenters asked their subjects to recognize the scene and the emotion portrayed. The exposure length was cut again and again to see at what point accuracy was diminished. Even at an exposure of 1/24 of a second, people were correct over two thirds of the time.

NONVERBAL BEHAVIOR OF THE PATIENT

Effective communicators have long understood the salience of nonverbal communication to their work. All experienced health professionals know that a verbally silent client is still communicating a great deal of information at the nonverbal level. Even highly verbal clients express much more than just their words. As Erickson and colleagues (1976) have stated, "a person seeking therapy comes in and tells you one story that is believed fully at the conscious level and in nonverbal language can give you a story that is entirely different." Successful family therapists will observe the spatial arrangement chosen by patients and watch carefully for nonverbal cues as the family members interact. Recently one of the authors worked with a married couple in which the wife complained of feeling tense and angry a great deal of the time without understanding why. She finally became aware of the many nonverbal cues her husband communicated that irritated her. For example, he often looked away and grimaced in a frustrating manner when she spoke. He also displayed a very subtle patronizing gesture with his hands when she was angry, and her anger only increased as a result. This woman was not conscious of her reactions to these nonverbal signals. Since it so often bypasses the analytical and rational processes of the conscious mind, nonverbal communication can exert a powerful influence upon human behavior.

Many health professionals generate some preliminary hypotheses or opinions about a patient even before words are spoken. The clothes worn, the gait and posture displayed, the tonal quality of the voice, the color and muscle tone of the face are all cues that communicate a great deal. All health professionals can increase their effectiveness by being open to nonverbal cues. Furthermore, steps can be taken to open up sensory channels to better pace a patient. If you already have evidence that, like most people, you use one representational system more than another (see Chapter 3), you can consciously begin to pay more attention to cues from the other systems. If your primary system has been visual, concentrate on audition and be more attentive to what your patient says and how he or she says it. A common complaint of patients is that "my doctor doesn't *hear* what I'm saying." If your primary system is auditory, pay closer attention to your patients' visual cues; concentrate on movements and gestures of the body, especially subtle changes in muscle tone and color of the face. You *can* open up your sensory channels with concentration and practice. And sooner than you think, you will be pleasantly surprised to find that you will automatically or unconsciously be more open to a variety of cues and therefore begin to communicate more effectively.

ELICITING AND USING "YES" AND "NO" CUES

A valuable strategy for the health professional is to become more aware of the patient's nonverbal signals for communicating "yes" and "no." In order to illustrate a procedure to accomplish this, silently answer the following questions: (1) At this very moment are you reading these words? (2) Would you like to be a more effective health professional? (3) Do you enjoy being happy? (4) Have you ever been unhappy? Now answer these questions: (1) Do you like being unhappy? (2) Are you eight years old or younger? (3) Is this the third time that you have read this book? (4) Would you like to serve time in a prison? Now try to be aware of nonverbal signals for "yes" and for "no" that you emitted when you answered the first four questions and the last four questions. For example, for yes, did you nod your head, gesture with a finger or hand or foot, or move your lips subtly in some particular way? For no, did you shake your head back and forth or move some other finger or your hand or foot or lips in a particular way? Or perhaps your movements were even more subtle, such as a mild cock of the head or a shifting of the eyes. All of these patterns are commonly used as nonverbal and often unconscious signals.

It is standard practice for most health professionals to ask a patient a variety of questions at an initial interview. If this has not been your practice, incorporating some "yes" and "no" questions into your initial communication with a patient can be quite simple (e.g., "It's a beautiful day today, isn't it?" or "Do you have these headaches every day?"). Closely observe your patient's nonverbal cues for "yes" and "no," and you have established a valuable resource to enhance your effectiveness.

You may ask, What is the purpose of learning to read these nonverbal cues when you could just ask the patient the yes and no questions? Well, the answer is both obvious and complicated. Since we believe that people respond from both the conscious and unconscious parts of themselves, we know that the answers are not always similar. It is therefore possible to read whether the person is totally congruent with what he or she is saying or whether he or she is in conflict by using nonverbal cues. For example if a person responding to your questions tells you he is not feeling any better and yet gives you nonverbal cues that he is, you then have information about the person's conflict (probably meaning that there are secondary gains about getting better, in this case). An effective professional will then use this information in working with the client.

Here is another illustration of how nonverbal cues can be utilized for effective communication. Implicit in the idea of pacing (see Chapter 2) is that patients are not always ready for just any information to be communicated to them at any moment. We can assume that only the experience or data that patients are willing to accept will be successfully incorporated by them. Otherwise there will be resistance to data communicated, and the health professional increases the probability of losing some credibility. Knowledge of your patients' unconscious nonverbal cues for "yes" and "no" can help you to pace your patients and be more effective.

Dr. Golden, a skilled communicator and an effective dentist, has just finished examining his patient, Mr. Smith. As Mr. Smith, a very quiet person, gets up from the dental chair, Dr. Golden says, "At this point, it is important for us to make an appointment for a root canal procedure." As he speaks, Dr. Golden observes Mr. Smith shake his head slightly (a nonverbal sign for "no"). Mr. Smith also pinches the bottom of his nostrils with the thumb and index finger of a hand. This is a common nonverbal signal for "it smells" or "I dislike." Immediately, Dr. Golden places his hand on Mr. Smith's shoulder (Mr. Smith is very kinesthetic) and says, "However, I have a feeling that you may need some more information. So let's sit down in my office, go over what we've done so far, and I think you'll have a better grasp of all this real soon." After communicating more information to Mr. Smith and perceiving "yes" signals from him, Dr. Golden successfully suggests another appointment for the root canal procedure.

Health professionals are commonly confronted with situations in which there are multiple solutions or treatment strategies available for a clinical problem. In these situations, a sensitivity to the patient's nonverbal signals for "yes" and "no" can be very helpful. Dr. Jones, an orthopedic surgeon, is speaking to her patient, Mrs. Myers, who has been in bed for several weeks with lower back pain and some pain and numbness in her right leg. Dr. Jones tells her patient that the symptoms are suggestive of a disc problem and that Mrs. Myers has these options available to her: (1) hospitalization with pelvic traction, (2) further diagnostic procedures such as a myelogram, which would cause some discomfort, and (3) calling in a neurosurgeon for a consultation. Mrs. Myers responds with a great deal of confusion and indecisiveness. Dr. Jones then goes over each detail, answering all questions from Mrs. Myers. Dr. Jones carefully observes the reactions of her patient and observes that Mrs. Myers appears tense and sounds slightly more anxious when asking for more information for alternatives one and three. Dr. Jones then states that she would like Mrs. Myers to decide on an alternative and repeats them one last time. As she repeats each one, she observes that Mrs. Myers shakes her head very slightly as alternatives one and three are mentioned and that Mrs. Myers nods her head slightly when alternative two is mentioned. Mrs. Myers again expresses her indecisiveness and states, "What do you suggest, Doctor? I want you to decide." At that point, Dr. Jones recommends alternative two and Mrs. Myers expresses satisfaction (verbally and nonverbally) with the decision.

Reading nonverbal cues requires practice. However, there is something you can do now that will prove to be immediately beneficial and will also serve as a tool for practicing your observational skills. What we suggest is that you learn to trust your skill, which you already unconsciously possess, in noticing other people's unconscious messages. Sometimes in a patient interaction one gets a vague feeling that the patient is not listening or is not going to follow directions. The health professional may not consciously notice that the patient's head shook slightly, or that the eyes shifted downward, or that the shoulders tensed at a particular moment. All the health professional knows is that there seems to be a strong feeling that the patient either did not absorb the input or is not going to follow it. As we have discussed in previous chapters, this feeling is based on a specific unconscious recognition of minute perceptual data that are being received. What we ask you to do is to utilize these unconscious resources both by noticing your feelings in these situations and by acting on them accordingly.

S.G., a physical therapist at a Pittsburgh hospital, incorporates these principles into his work beautifully. He realizes that the work the patient does between visits is extremely important both for the actual physical aspect of conditioning and for the patient's sense of self-responsibility. He therefore always leaves adequate time at the end of each session to cover the homework assignments for the patient. He tells us that he never finishes with patients if he has a feeling that they will not do the assigned tasks for the week. He will first mention the suggested homework and then spend time explaining why it needs to be done. With many of his patients the nonverbal behavior does not communicate that the patient will necessarily comply, so he repeats the whole thing again in different words. Sometimes he repeats the same message five or six times in various ways, often using indirect communication techniques (these will be discussed in Chapter 6). He always makes sure that before he finishes with the patient he has a definite positive feeling that the patient will complete the homework instructions.

So far, our discussion has focused on the nonverbal behavior of the patient. We have stressed the importance of the health professional observing and utilizing these cues in order to enhance communication effectiveness. Our discussion will now turn to an area of at least equal importance: the role of the nonverbal behavior and patterns of the health professional in creative and effective communication.

NONVERBAL BEHAVIOR OF THE HEALTH PROFESSIONAL

Just as the nonverbal behavior of patients can communicate so much, the same is true for the health professional. Your patient is keenly aware, consciously or unconsciously, of much more than what you say. In fact, since patients are usually experiencing some kind of hurt, pain, or discomfort when they seek help, they are very likely to be particularly sensitive to many aspects of your behavior.

In Chapter 2, the idea of congruence in behavior was presented. Effective communication is congruent. This means that verbal and nonverbal aspects of the communicator's behavior are consistent; bodily movements and tone of voice will all reflect the verbal message. Think of effective and famous communicators such as Billy Graham, and it is quickly apparent how all elements of his behavior mirror his words. When preaching, Billy Graham communicates as much or more with his body and voice tonality as with his words. If his message is gentle, he will hold a finger to his lips and whisper. If his words are angry, he will shout as his fists pound the podium. His audience is left with little doubt that Billy Graham is earnest and sincerely believes what he says and as such is influenced by him.

We so often hear that patients "know what's really going on" when it comes to their condition; therefore, we should be truthful with them. Translated this statement means that patients are sensitive to other cues besides our words. A tense voice tone and a gaze away from your patient's eyes as you say that "everything will be all right" may cause confusion and distress. If you have determined that it is not appropriate to be absolutely truthful with a patient, saying nothing at all may be preferred.

At times, stress from your personal life can carry over into your professional work. Because patients are sensitive to our nonverbal behavior they can perceive this stress and misinterpret it. Mrs. Black, a registered nurse, graduated from nursing school about six months ago. She works on a ward for acutely ill patients in a general hospital. Mrs. Black is usually a very cheerful, friendly person. However, several weeks ago she began to have distressful marital problems. She tried to maintain a "happy face," but her patients and fellow colleagues perceived nonverbal cues of stress and unhappiness and were distressed by the incongruence in her behavior. A few patients asked Mrs. Black if their own condition had deteriorated or if tests they took indicated that anything was wrong. Some of her colleagues asked Mrs. Black if she was angry with them. Finally, her supervisor asked to meet with her, and Mrs. Black disclosed that she had been having problems at home but that fortunately she was resolving them. At her supervisor's suggestion, Mrs. Black shared with some of her patients and colleagues that she was having some personal problems, but that she was effectively handling them. She immediately noticed that her patients and colleagues felt better because they understood what had been going on. She herself felt more comfortable. Interestingly, some of her patients gave some encouragement and support, which seemed to "perk" them up. As this example illustrates, many health professionals have discovered that at times it is desirable and appropriate to engage in some self-disclosing behavior because patients may perceive incongruent nonverbal behavior. It can help the health professional to be more comfortable in the clinical situation and therefore to increase his or her effectiveness.

Many times a health professional may want to request that a client recall certain past experiences. For example, we often ask our patients to remember a time from their past (either a recent past or a distant past) when they felt really good about themselves; when they felt really powerful and potent. This is often important because sometimes in times of crisis we all lose touch with the personal power that each of us has and that can be used to help us in troubled times. It is very difficult to help a person return to this state if the health professional sits back and in a very quiet monotone says to the patient, "Now I want you to remember a time when you felt very powerful." The patient is helped immensely in re-experiencing such a state if the health professional sits up (or even stands up), is animated, raises his voice, and says the same words.

So far, we have discussed the importance of congruence in verbal and nonverbal behavior for effective communication. Let us now briefly discuss some other important aspects of nonverbal communication.

NONVERBAL PACING

This concept, discussed in depth in Chapter 2, bears repeating because of its importance for effective communication. Nonverbal pacing involves mirroring one or more aspects of the patient's nonverbal behavior. It is most effective when it is done subtly or beyond the patient's conscious awareness. An important type of nonverbal pacing is breathing at the same rate as the patient. Other forms of nonverbal pacing include mirroring a patient's body posture, gestures, and voice tone, tempo, and amplitude. One of the authors recently had an experience that illustrates the effectiveness of nonverbal pacing. He was asked to see a 25-year-old vocational rehabilitation client who was severely paralyzed on the left side and who was a serious stutterer. The patient could only whisper words very quietly and even then only when accompanied by a ritualistic type of straining and gesturing of the upper part of his body. It was obvious that his vocal cords locked severely when he attempted to speak, a common element of stuttering. The client communicated primarily through the use of a crude form of sign language and by writing notes. It was known that this client was shot in the head earlier in his life, which produced organic damage and the resulting paralysis. However, no organic reasons for his mutism or stuttering were ever found, and this symptom was diagnosed as being psychogenic and a result of the trauma of being shot. Numerous health professionals had been unable to obtain details from this client as to the circumstances of the shooting that injured him. He was labeled as being "highly resistant."

The patient was accompanied to the author's office by his vocational rehabilitation counselor, who desired a psychological evaluation of the client. The author immediately paced many of the patient's behaviors. The patient's stooped posture and breathing rate were mirrored. The author also mirrored the patient's straining, gesturing, and whispering as the two communicated. Within minutes, the author learned from the patient that at the age of ten he was accidentally shot by his own brother while both were playing with a gun. In 15 years no health professional had been able to obtain this information. Within a few minutes, the patient was talking a little more loudly and cooperating enthusiastically. The vocational rehabilitation counselor was amazed.

TOUCHING

Touch may be the most important of all nonverbal behaviors. We are all familiar with the critical importance of touch to human development. A severe deprivation of touching during infancy and childhood can produce serious psychopathological conditions. In the past, touch was considered so powerful and therapeutic that cures were attempted (and were no doubt successful in many cases) by the "laying on of hands." Such acts continue to be used in many cultures today.

In most health professions touching is a frequent occurrence and a vital means of communication. Nurses touch a patient when taking a temperature or a blood pressure or when giving an injection. Physicians touch during an examination; dentists and physical therapists obviously touch to perform their work. X-ray technicians often touch patients when preparing them for a series of x-rays. Touching communicates a great deal about your caring and sensitivity for the patient. Patients will often express a preference for a particular physician or dentist because of that person's "gentle touch."

Technology, however, may be jeopardizing the important therapeutic value of touch. In her text, *Behavioral Concepts and the Critically Ill Patient* (1976), Sharon L. Roberts illustrates this point:

> In today's highly technical hospital environment, dominated by machines, the patient loses precedence to the machines. The patient then experiences technological deprivation. With technological deprivation comes emotional deprivation. For example, a patient in ICU may be surrounded by various pieces of equipment: a cardioscope, a chest tube and gomco suction, IVs and a respirator. (As the nurse comes to the patient's bed, she approaches his equipment first; when the equipment is checked, she then looks at the patient.) This is a correct nursing response: she must run rhythm strips, check dial settings, rate of IV solution, and carry out other procedures. After gathering her data, the nurse will move toward her patient and, possibly, touch him, but she has given more nursing care time to the various machines than to her patient. The nurse cannot be faulted for this because she must fill the squares on her patient's chart with numbers and words at the designated time. She has patient responsibilities, her time is limited, she must gather her data and move on to the next patient. Day nurses must put all their data in order before the parade of doctors and technicians begins.

Many health professionals have ambivalent or, in some cases, negative feelings about touching. Usually such attitudes reflect taboos from childhood carried over into adulthood. Sometimes there is conflict and confusion; for example, many people incorrectly equate touching with overt sexuality. The authors have met health professionals who refuse to touch any patients unless absolutely necessary because "they may accuse me of seductive behavior." Some patients may indeed misinterpret touching as a sexual overture. But in many cases, it is the health professional's own attitudes that are getting in the way. It would be wise for all of us to examine and explore exactly what our attitudes about touching are. Answering the following questions can be helpful: (1) Do you ever touch a patient to express affection or caring? (2) Do you feel more free to touch a child than an adult patient? (3) Do you feel more comfortable touching persons of one sex or of one race more than the other?

Jim, a beginning counselor in a family services agency, expressed frustration to his supervisor. He said that several patients became very teary-eyed when he talked with them and he didn't know whether or not he should keep on talking with them. His supervisor asked Jim if he ever felt like responding in other ways at such moments. Jim said he sometimes wanted to touch or embrace the patients but felt too anxious about that. He was told to take the risk to do "what his senses told him to do" with a few select patients. At his next supervisory session, Jim reported that he touched one patient's hand and they had a very productive session. He touched another teary-eyed patient on the shoulder and then embraced that person, who cried a great deal. This patient made important emotional breakthroughs during the session and Jim reported that he also learned a great deal from the encounter.

Touching may be an especially effective means of communication for patients whose primary representational system is kinesthetic (see Chapter 3). A touch or embrace is a common and usually positive and comforting kinesthetic cue or anchor established during childhood. Using such anchors can be helpful in many clinical situations (see Chapter 8).

As with all forms of communication, touch is most effective when used at the appropriate time and place. For example, some persons may at times consider touching an invasion of their privacy or personal space. There are many occasions when the health professional must rely on clinical judgment as to when to engage in tactile communication.

SPACE

Space is a multifaceted dimension of nonverbal communication. It can refer to the personal or private invisible space around our bodies. Such personal space varies from individual to individual. Some people feel comfortable only a few inches away from another person. Other people may feel uneasy unless there is a distance of at least four or five feet between themselves and someone else. Generally, two or three feet or less can be considered an intimate distance.

Some health professionals such as nurses, physicians, dentists, and physical therapists must, of necessity, be involved with patients at intimate distances. Since some patients will be uncomfortable with this closeness, it is important to be aware of nonverbal cues of anxiety or discomfort and to respond in some way that will comfort the patient. Some gentle words at these times can be very helpful, such as "I know that some people get uncomfortable in situations like this, but we'll be through in just a minute or two." This immediately paces the ongoing experience of discomfort so that the professional can begin leading the clients toward greater ease.

Some health professionals, such as social workers, will often not be in the intimate proximity of their patients. During an initial interview, these health professionals will usually be seated at a comfortable distance from the patient. Thereafter, they can rely on their own clinical judgment and awareness of the nonverbal cues of the patient as to what the intimacy of the meeting warrants. There may be moments—for example, when a patient is tearful or crying—when it is best to move into close proximity of the patient. Oftentimes, of course, crying may be used for a manipulative purpose and at these times it may be advantageous to keep one's distance.

Space can also refer to the concept of "territoriality." This is the common tendency to stake out territory—both space and things—and call it our own. Marion Blondis and Barbara Jackson, in their text *Nonverbal Communication With Patients* (1977), discuss how territorial space and things are especially important to hospitalized patients:

> When a patient is checked into the hospital, territorial things and space are left behind. The day before he checks into the hospital, he has a clear identity, which is reinforced by all of his territorial surroundings. Suddenly, the night before surgery he finds himself in unfamiliar, often frightening, surroundings, wearing an embarrassing hospital gown. He was probably cautioned to leave his wallet, jewelry, and credit cards at home. There is no territorial reinforcement. He has ceased to be John Jones, the most successful plumber in East Hamden, Ohio. He

has become, instead, Dr. Smith's gall bladder case. It is all routine for us, but it is not for him. A little empathy for his nervousness might go a long way toward helping him through the next day's ordeal.

Long-term patients have special problems in relating to their hospital environment. For example, an elderly patient in a skilled nursing facility suddenly lost her husband. She mourned terribly and developed the habit of opening a small box of memorabilia kept in her bedside stand, strewing the contents all over her bed—pictures, bits of ribbon, old letters, and other souvenirs. One of the staff nurses would catch her, scold her for being so messy, carefully pack everything into the box and pop it back into the night stand. The elderly lady would try and dig the box out again as soon as the nurse's back was turned. The nurse did not recognize that the box of memorabilia was the old woman's last tie with her territory—with all that was her life.

Communicating one's sensitivity to a patient's territory can often be done nonverbally. For example, knocking on the hospital room door (when possible) before entering, or gently handling clothing or other possessions will be appreciated.

TIME

Can you remember when you felt angry or frustrated because you were kept waiting by someone? Such experiences immediately remind us how time can be a potent dimension of nonverbal communication. A patient kept waiting by a health professional may perceive this as disrespect or insensitivity. Extra time spent with patients is usually perceived as indicative of an attitude of caring and interest. What may be communicated if you are glancing anxiously at your watch as you sit with a patient is obvious.

All health professionals are aware of how much can be communicated by the variable of time. For example, patients who consistently arrive late for psychotherapy may be nonverbally, and often unconsciously, communicating that they are angry at the therapist or anxious about their treatment. Most experienced therapists have been confronted with patients who regularly begin to ask questions or get into something "heavy" when the time is near for their session to be over. Quite often such patients are nonverbally asking, "Do you care enough about me to spend more time with me?" Such situations must be handled by the therapist sensitively. Often the correct strategy is to insist on stopping the session on time. This (nonverbally) can communicate limits and boundaries to the patient.

This chapter has discussed the importance of nonverbal communication for health professionals. A sensitivity to the nonverbal cues of patients and an awareness of your own nonverbal communication can significantly increase your effectiveness. To demonstrate to you the power of both observing other people's nonverbal behavior and consciously communicating nonverbally to others, we'd like to end this chapter by telling you how we start the many workshops we teach for health professionals on this topic. Before we start the group, we pick out someone we do not know in the audience by watching their nonverbal behaviors, such as watching where they sit (usually picking someone fairly close to the front and to the center), noticing their alertness and their attentiveness level, and seeing them interact with other people (so that we know that they will not be extremely shy in front of a group). We then write down on a piece of paper a description of this person. We walk in and start the workshop by sitting down in the front of the room with an empty chair between us. As we walk in, we put the piece of paper with the person's description on it under the empty chair. We then stare at the group for five to ten minutes. This is done for two reasons. First, it establishes attentiveness as the group sits curious and sometimes anxious about what we are going to do. Second, it establishes our authority over the group, because as we make eye contact with them it is usually more comfortable for us than for most of the group participants. What we also do, however, is to invite the chosen group participant to come to the front of the room and sit in the empty chair. We do this by making much more contact with him or her than with the rest of the group in the room. After we catch this person's gaze, we shift our eyes very subtly to the empty chair and occasionally nod our heads very slightly in an up-and-down direction. After the silence is over, we start the group by asking, "Will the person who's going to be the first demonstration subject please come up to this chair." We then proceed to open the group with a demonstration of one of our communication techniques. Over the past three years over 80 per cent of the time the first person to come up has been the person we nonverbally invited to do so. The nonverbal invitations we give are so subtle that whenever we ask the person why they came up, the answers were always conscious reasons such as, "I knew I'd want to do it, so I thought I'd get it over with instead of pressing myself for the next two days," or "One of my friends who was in a workshop previously said it was a very interesting experience to do." We have never had a participant verbalize to us their awareness of our maneuvers. They are always quite surprised and even happy when we ask them at the end of this demonstration to bend down and pick up the piece of paper under the chair and they see a description of themselves. One important element needs to be added here. After this demonstration we always thank the person profusely for being so open at the unconscious level that he or she was willing to communicate with us. In this way, we label this openness a good trait of the subject's as opposed to making it seem as though we have power over them.

EXERCISES

1. Break up into small groups and take turns playing the roles of communicator and subject while the other group members act as observers. The communicator should ask the subject five obvious "yes" and five obvious "no" questions and closely observe the subject's nonverbal cues. Now ask the subject a series of questions for which you don't know the answers while the subject answers "yes" or "no" silently to himself (e.g., "Do you have an older brother?" or "Do you like football?"). Keeping in mind the nonverbal cues you observed earlier, guess whether the answer is "yes" or "no."
2. Break up into groups of three and take turns playing the following three roles: A, B, and C. A remembers a past experience that was very emotional (happiness, joy, fear, anger) and nonverbally portrays what he or she is experiencing. B observes closely A's behavior and nonverbally paces the behavior. C then guesses the emotion or emotions being experienced. Discuss the experience.

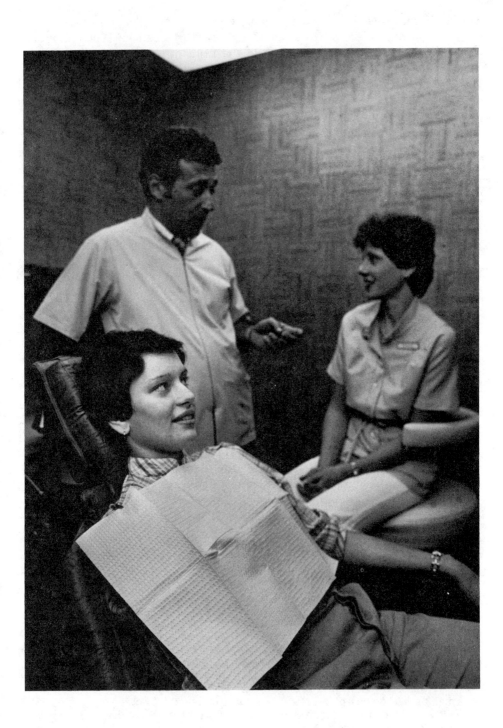

Indirect Communication 6

Unlike the direct forms of communication discussed in Chapter 4, in which it is obvious to the patient what the health professional is attempting to communicate, the messages and the processes of giving information discussed in this chapter are often hidden in terms of both the intent and the possible power of the message. There are basically two major reasons that health professionals might sometimes want to use indirect communication techniques with their clients. The primary reason for using these techniques is that many times they are clearly the most effective communication techniques that a health professional can use. The reason for their effectiveness is that, if done well, these types of messages can tap into the unconscious resources of the patient. This is in contrast to direct forms of communication, which are almost exclusively limited to the patient's consciousness. In the introduction to this text we have already stated why we believe it is important for a health professional, or any effective communicator, to have an open channel to the receiver's unconscious. To restate, before most patients come to a health professional, they have already tried to use their own conscious resources to solve their problems. These attempts have mostly been unsuccessful, otherwise the health professional would not need any special techniques to get his or her messages across. An example would be the young man facing the physical therapist without having practiced his exercises for the week. You could probably assume that the young man has talked to himself and has probably received pep talks from his parents and doctor, who have futilely attempted to get him to practice the exercises. We do not believe it is useful for the health professional, in this case the physical therapist, to become one more person fighting or negotiating with the consciousness of this particular client. Such a tack, which is the one that is most usually taken is more often than not doomed to failure.

Unfortunately, most of the communication courses taught in a university (particularly in the schools attended by health professionals) and most of the models that health professionals see in action limit the response possibilities to those types of responses that communicate with the left side of the brain, or the conscious mind of the patient. Sometimes such communication techniques are very effective. But please note: the key word in the previous sentence is sometimes. Health professionals who have methods for gaining access to the unconscious resources of their patients will have more options when trying to decide what would be the most effective way for them to communicate a particular message to a particular client at a particular time. This goes back to one of the key concepts of the first chapter—flexibility, or requisite variety. The more requisite variety that communicators have, the greater the possibility they have of being successful at actualizing the intent of their communications.

A second very important reason for studying and occasionally using indirect forms of communication is that this process of communication often keeps the health professional much more interested and alert to all the possibilities of communication. Boredom and burn-out are two "B's" not fully explored in many schools of medicine, dentistry, nursing, and allied health. But there are only so many cavities you can fill, depressed patients you can talk to, or noncompliant patients that you might work with before you begin to get bored with the entire healing process. Suddenly you find yourself working more for money or out of habit than for the original ideas and goals that you had when you first entered your profession. There's a prima facie case for believing that a bored professional will not do as good a job on any given patient as a professional with the same degree of training and experience who is still interested in the healing process. Creating and using new forms of direct and particularly indirect communication techniques will help the clinician stay alert to his or her patient, since all effective communication has to pace each individual patient. The health professional will be more interested in the healing process and, more importantly, will feel like a creative professional rather than a technician.

The choice of whether for a particular patient at any given moment a direct, straightforward suggestion or one of the many forms of indirect communication aimed at the patient's unconscious is appropriate needs to be based on the clinical judgment of the individual practitioner. Before making judgments about the appropriateness of any given method, one needs to have experience in that method and confidence in the ability to adequately employ it. Thus, clinical judgments are not based on ignorance or on the fear of failure.

Many of the methods to be discussed in this chapter may at first seem silly, inappropriate, or possibly even unprofessional. In particular, it will seem as though it should be very easy for the patient to see through your actions and understand your intent. We suggest that you use these methods often enough to feel comfortable with them and to make an accurate assessment about whether they might be useful at some time for you. This often requires taking a psychological risk. Trying them one at a time or in mild versions can minimize the risk. The authors all know how powerful these skills are; but none of us knew it when we first started. We were all lucky enough to observe some very effective communicators use these techniques. Because of these observations, we were willing to take the risk and try new methods. Subsequently, we have all become much more effective communicators than when we were limited to the more traditional methods of trying to get a message across. *You* will never know if any of these techniques are as powerful as we claim until *you* are also willing to take some risks and to grow a little as a health professional.

Probably the most elegant form of indirect communication is the use of metaphors and stories, which we will examine in the next chapter. The remainder of this chapter will consist of some description, with clinical examples, of simpler and yet extremely powerful and effective indirect communication techniques. It will become obvious to you as you read on that these techniques overlap quite a bit with each other. The techniques are actually only given to you as examples of a process. The variety of such techniques is limited only by the imagination of the communicator. Some of these are standard techniques that we use and teach to our students and that you might find helpful to experiment with. Hopefully, when you find the process of indirect communication as successful as we believe you will, you will begin experimenting with different area of the skills we talk about. In fact, you'll invent many techniques on your own as you begin more and more to trust your own "intuition," which is probably the best clinical tool you have at your disposal.

The last major advantage of the indirect communication techniques that we will discuss is that they do not require a reply (often a defensive reply) by the client. We all know that the person who is interested in telling the best joke at a party doesn't hear the other jokes because he's too busy thinking of his own during the conversation. All human beings have a need to publicly defend themselves. Once a patient has done something that the health professional doesn't like, such as not taking medication, not staying on an exercise regimen, or creating a problem for a nurse in the hospital, it is very hard for the patient to fully recoup and cooperate with the health professional, since often the response is in some way one of chastisement. You will notice that the techniques that we're about to elaborate most often do not require any reply on the part of the subject. Therefore, even though the patient knows you're talking about him or her, at an unconscious level and sometimes in a way even at a conscious level, the patient has the option of pretending (just as you are) that you're really talking about someone or something else. This allows the patient to fully hear what you say at both a conscious and an unconscious level and to respond accordingly without giving up "personhood" and integrity in the process.

USE OF TELEPHONE

One of the most effective and least expensive co-workers that any health professional can have is the weather person provided to you courtesy of the telephone company. By using the telephone, you can look a patient straight in the eye and say exactly what you want to tell him or her. You can do it under the pretense of talking to another client or co-worker. In this way, the patient is able to absorb consciously and unconsciously your entire message, without having to become defensive and respond verbally to you.

As a strategy worked out in conjunction with the physicians, a nurse-practitioner working the reception room in the office of a pediatric team picked up the telephone as a particular mother came into the waiting room and up to her desk. This mother was a problem for the physicians and the nurse-practitioner, since she was the kind of mother who ran her child to the pediatrician once or twice a week for what seemed like every possible little hangnail or blackhead. The nurse-practitioner spoke into the telephone and said—as she looked directly at the mother—"No, Mrs. Jones, we can't fit you right in today or tomorrow because you come here much too often on a so-called emergency basis and keep disrupting our schedule. They really are minor ailments that by this time you should be able to handle by yourself. It is really going to become important for you to learn to distinguish between those things that you need our help with and those you don't. Why don't you call Dr. Smith tomorrow between eight and nine during his calling hours and he can talk to you for a few minutes to help you with your problem. Okay, good-bye." With that she hung up the phone and then took the questions of the mother who had come into the office. This mother, at some level, will understand that part of that message was directed at her and will be able to incorporate that into her own thought processes. Yet she was able to receive the message without having been embarrassed by the nurse-practitioner or pediatrician and without having to respond in some kind of defensive or face-saving way.

Some of the health professionals or students reading this book may also be or become teachers. Here is a very clear recent example where one of the authors used a variation of the telephone technique. A student had made an appointment to come to his office and the professor knew clearly that the student was going to ask for an incomplete, as this was her habit throughout her whole graduate studies. The professor decided not to give her an incomplete, but at this time did not feel it was appropriate nor did he desire to take the time and energy to confront the student with her behavior. It also would have been redundant, as other teachers had done the same thing previously. As the student walked down the hall and approached the office, the author dialed the weather and while talking into the phone (the student being able to hear very faintly another voice on the other end), the professor looked right at the student as she walked to the door of his office and said into the telephone, "No, I'm sorry, Melissa (not the student's name), I'm not going to give you an incomplete. You've already had two from me and it's not fair to the other students in the class. I understand that some life situations are presently tough for you, but you're going to have to do the best you can to get the paper in on time. I'm sorry. Good-bye." The professor then looked up and greeted the student at the door, whereupon she spent two or three minutes of his time asking a face-saving trivial question that she probably would never have made an appointment to ask and then left the office. The student got the message and yet was not embarrassed; the professor was able to do what he wanted to do in the situation without having to spend time dealing with a crying, pleading student in his office. Sometimes it is very important and appropriate to be straightforward and direct. Sometimes that style is not effective for your patients or you. Just as with all other tools of your trade, an individual clinical judgment needs to be made.

A child development worker wanted to give a 7-year-old child a magic rock that came from an old Indian who lived in the hills of Arizona. She wanted to establish the magical powers of this rock, which would help the child deal with some of the fears he had about being alone in certain parts of his house. Therefore the child development worker, while working with the child, had her secretary call up in the middle of the session. The worker picked up the phone and said into it, "Oh James, I'm glad to hear that. I didn't think you'd be finished with it for another week or so, but since it's worked already, I wish you would bring it back to me when you come in tomorrow. I have another friend that I want to give it to who could use it right now also. Okay, good-bye, see you tomorrow, thanks." The child development worker put the telephone down and turned excitedly to the child in her office. She told him about the magic rock she had that she had intended to surprise him with. Since she was going to get it back tomorrow, the next time he came in she would have it available. She even took down the picture that she had in her office of the mountain in Arizona and pointed out exactly where the rock came from and told a little about its history. (By the way, if you don't believe in magic rocks, it's probably very difficult for you to work with children.)

TALKING ABOUT OR TO SOMEONE ELSE

One of the most effective ways to communicate to patients is to talk, in their presence, to someone else about them or about someone else, or even to talk directly to them about someone else. Some of the most effective health professionals hardly ever say anything to the patients about themselves but almost always talk about the patient who just left.

One of the authors is somewhat lazy and not as health oriented in some areas for himself as he should be. For years his dentist, whom he knew personally, had tried to get him to floss his teeth. The dentist talked, pleaded, yelled, and showed all kind of horror films and pictures, all to no avail. One visit, after the hygienist had cleaned the author's teeth, the dentist came in for his routine check to see if there were any cavities. When looking at the gums, he turned to the hygienist and casually said, "I don't think he has to go to the periodontist *yet*." This author has flossed his teeth every day since that incident, which happened close to a year ago.

A family therapist was working with a family in which the father kept interrupting everyone, particularly the mother. One time when the mother was discussing a very important personal issue, the father again interrupted. As every family systems person discovers somewhere along the line, this process will need to be pointed out consciously to the family and they will have to work on it. But at this time the therapist did not want to interrupt the mother once again, even if it was to point out this process. What the therapist did was to sigh, sit back in the chair for a minute, take a sip of his Pepsi, and say, "I'm sorry, I seem exhausted today but I'm glad that you're such a good family to work with because the family before you was such a problem. The father kept interrupting everyone. I finally had to say to him"—at which time the therapist looks directly at the father—"if you don't stop interrupting you're going to have to leave.'" Certainly everyone in the family, except the father, understood what the message was about. You could see by the twinkle in their eyes. And certainly the father understood at one level because he kept quiet and let the mother do what she needed to do. However, the father was not embarrassed or forced to defend himself in front of his family, which would have taken the time and energy that the therapist did not want to take at this particular moment. So for this particular occasion, this was a very effective communication in that the therapist accomplished what he wanted and yet did it with minimal embarrassment or interruption to the process or to the family.

A physician in family practice had a client come in who seemed particularly reluctant to take important medication. The physician tried logically explaining and even getting angry with the client, to no avail. Since this physician had a considerable amount of requisite variety, he was able to get the client to change his behavior by saying to the client one day as he walked in (after using his sensory channels and once again just being able to see by the skin tone and demeanor of the patient that the medication had not been taken regularly), "I'm sorry if I'm in a rotten mood today but it just really annoys me that his patient who I've had for a long time and whom I really like a lot was just in here a half hour ago and he has refused to follow my directions about some medications and he's just about on the verge of having to go to the hospital. He has some really serious things wrong with him and I'm very frustrated that I can't get him to do what needs to be done. Since I like you too, I'm glad that you're beginning to listen and take your medicine." This not only got across the message about the seriousness of the patient's condition to him, but the physician also set up a self-fulfilling prophecy by saying, "I know you're a good patient and you're taking your medicine."

A final example of the effectiveness of talking to one person about another person follows. A 17-year-old teenager, mother of two children, had presented to the hospital with abdominal pain and fever. The doctor started her on intravenous antibiotics because of a presumed diagnosis of pelvic infection. After several days, the patient continued to spike a high temperature daily. Because of this clinical picture, the presence of pelvic abscess was considered. A laparotomy was suggested to search for this abscess. One of the nurses on the floor thought that the patient might be putting the thermometer under hot water to simulate a fever. As the abdominal pain had now resolved, this seemed to be a likely possibility. After closely observing her each time she had the thermometer over the next 24 hours, the nurse reported that there was no more fever. The patient, however, totally denied interfering with the thermometer. The physician and nurse obviously deemed it very important to learn the truth, since the fever could have recurred at any time if it was not factitious. With repeated questioning, the patient continued to deny everything, although her nonverbal behavior was not congruent with this denial.

At this point the nurse decided to tell a simple story. She told her about "Mrs. Rodman" over on Four-North, who had been a patient three and a half months previously. She had come into the hospital very sick and with a high fever. After about a week the staff found out that she had been dipping her thermometer under hot water and thus faking her fever. The nurses and doctors asked why she had done this. She responded that she felt she was very sick but was afraid that they wouldn't find out what was wrong with her. She therefore pretended a fever so that they would have more time to find out what was really wrong with her. The nurse stated that when she and the doctor heard this they completely understood and weren't mad at all. After all, she was just trying to take care of herself to make sure she wouldn't die. How could they possibly fault her for this?

The wide-eyed patient looked up at the nurse and said, "You know, I did the same thing as that patient." After letting go of this, she then felt more open to talk about the events leading to her own hospitalization. For the next two minutes she revealed that she had thrown her 10-month-old child on the floor on its head several times in the previous week because she couldn't stand all the crying. She knew she just had to get out of her house. The abdominal pain had started at that time.

As you can see, these are just variations of the telephone method. Instead of talking to the weather lady or to your secretary, you talk directly to the patient or another health professional in the presence of the patient.

ILLUSION OF CHOICE

This method suggests that you give patients some choices that occupy their conscious mind, whereas the bottom line of any of the choices is that you— the health professional—get the patient to do what you want. This is a variation of the old parental trick of asking a child who they want to take a bath, "Do you want to take your bath before or after this television show?"

Two of the authors of this text are therapists who regularly practice clinical hypnosis. It's not uncommon for us to ask clients, "Do you want to sit in this chair and go into a trance or in that chair and go into a trance? Or, "Do you want to go into a light, medium, or deep trance today?" In the first instance, the patient's mind is occupied with the conscious choice of which chair looks more comfortable or which they're more used to and they end up making a choice by saying "this chair" of "that chair," usually without remembering consciously that the second half of the sentence is "and go into a trance." The second illusion of choice example is even more intriguing because none of us believes that the depth of trance really matters, since anyone will go into as deep a trance as they need in order to do their particular work (and we're not even sure that we or the patients know what it means to be in a light, medium, or deep trance anyway). So while the patient makes some decisions and has some feeling of being in control of the situation, they are still making a contract to go into a trance, which is what the intention of that particular communication was.

The medical technologist, coming in to draw blood from a patient believed to have a problem about this procedure, can come in smiling and say to the person, "Would you like my little pinch on your right arm or your left arm today?" Of course this message has two implications. The first is that the concept of "little pinch" is a positive way of letting the patient known it's not going to hurt much (if you remember, in the chapter on direct communication we suggested that you never say directly "This is not going to hurt much"). It also preoccupies the person consciously with a choice, that is, right arm or left arm, without fully realizing that when he makes the choice and says, "right arm," he's contracted for you to give that arm a "little pinch."

One of our students was a nurse who worked in a live-in rehabilitation center specializing in care for the elderly. She was working with a 60-year-old gentleman who was recuperating from an automobile accident much more slowly than the doctor thought was dictated by his physical condition. The nurse was an extremely effective communicator. After gaining his trust, she said to him one day, knowing that one of his major hobbies in life was betting on poker games and sporting events, "You know, we're taking a pool around here about when different people get better. I don't know if you know this about me, but Friday is my favorite day. It's the day I do all kinds of good things for myself. Since most of my patients like me, I find a lot of them, in fact most of them, get better also on Friday. We're starting to take a pool about when the first time you're going to walk for yourself will be. Now, I think it will be Friday because you like me and you're my patient and that's only three days from now. Of course, it's possible you could do it on Wednesday or Thursday, but I think it will be Friday. I guess it's even theoretically possible for you to do it Saturday or Sunday when I'm not here, but I'm confident you'll do it on Friday. Perhaps you'll wait another five, six days and do it on Monday or Tuesday, or even a whole week from now on next Wednesday, but . . . no . . . I'm pretty sure it will be on a Friday."

The basic choice she has given the patient is whether to be cooperative with her, in this case he'll start walking on Friday, or to show that he really is still under his own control, in which case he can walk any of the other days. He could even really spite her and do it on the weekend when she wasn't there. This method gives the client an active ability to outright resist what appears to be your desires, if that's what that particular patient needs to do in order to feel okay about himself. It also gives clients the choice for seeing themselves as the beautifully cooperative patient that some like to be. Of course, in this example, the nurse really didn't care which day this man started to walk. She would have been as happy on Wednesday as on Friday or Monday. The issue is that the patient gets caught up in the illusion that he's making an important choice by deciding the day and by deciding in a more indirect way whether he's going to be cooperative or not with his nurse. Yet the bottom line is that he is being motivated to get up and start walking at some day or another, which is all the health professional in this case really cared about. This is just a beautifully elegant example of effectively using illusion of choice (and also pacing the client's interest, in this case gambling), so that the health professional was able to use all of her clinical skills, linguistic as well as technological, to help this client do what he really needed to do for himself.

JUNKO LOGIC

Junko logic is a communication technique that very effective lawyer uses on a regular basis, especially while addressing a jury. It's the putting together of a group of facts, the first of which is indisputable and the last of which may be questionable; however, the goal of the statement is to get the receiver to believe the last fact. Let's suppose that in a law case facts X, Y, and Z are obvious and not disputable and fact A is in question. The lawyer would address the jury by saying that since X happened and Y and Z, then of Course A. The lawyer tries to show A as the logical outcome of X, Y, and Z, when in fact it may have no connection whatsoever.

A social worker we know starts off all his sessions with families by saying, "Since you're here today"—an indisputable fact easily verified by a census— "I know that you can do all the things you need to do to solve this problem." The second part of that statement becomes a kind of self-fulfilling prophecy after being associated with the first part of the statement, which has everyone thinking "yes."

A physical therapist might say to a person, "Since the muscles in your shoulders are getting much better developed," (if this in in fact the case and is clearly verifiable by the patient) "then it's going to become easier and easier for you to do exercise Y" (even if in fact exercise Y has nothing at all to do with the development of shoulder muscles).

By the way, since you are reading this book right now, we know that you are going to be a much more effective communicator even sooner than you think!

PARADOXICAL COMMANDS

Often, for one reason or another, you will get a patient who is into what we call polarity sets or responses, meaning that it seems they almost consistently do the opposite of what you ask of them. This is very often the case in working with adolescents who have a mental or physical health problem. Of course, once you recognize this phenomenon, if you are skilled at communication it is very easy to get these clients to do exactly what you want them to do for themselves.

One of the authors in private practice saw an adolescent girl brought in by her mother for enuresis. The parents had previously been to this psychologist for marriage counseling and in fact were seen by him as quite ineffective parents and in general quite ineffective people. When the oldest daughter was brought in to be treated, it became clear that she was in no way about to cooperate with the therapist, whom she saw as an authority figure aligned with her mother, another disliked authority figure. The family physician had explained to the mother and daughter that the problem was a "small bladder." This was a very strange diagnosis given the fact that every night the patient slept at home she urinated in her bed and that every night she slept at her girlfriend's, which during the summer was close to 50 per cent of the time, she never once urinated in her bed. (This is clearly a bladder whose size changes as the client walks in and out of the front door.) The mother was told that the therapist guaranteed a successful treatment if the mother followed the therapist's directions exactly, without one deviation and without asking questions. She was also told that the therapist would terminate treatment if, at any time, any of the instructions was not followed. The therapist then said to the patient in the privacy of his office, "I know that you're doing this to get back at your mother and I think you have every right to because your mother is a very ineffective mother. However, you're doing a half-assed job of it, and since I want your mother to get better because she is also my patient, I'm going to help you really get back at her." And so the therapist took out a prescription pad and wrote down the following: "Drink 8 oz. of water right before bed" the concession the child had made to her condition of a small bladder was not to drink an hour before bedtime); "sleep home every night" (this was a big thing to her because she liked to sleep at her girlfriend's house); and "pee in your bed every night." Of course, the client thought this was all a big joke and smiled and left after being told to come back next week for an appointment. The next week the family drove in to the therapist's office, which was over an hour from their house. The therapist kept them waiting in very uncomfortable quarters for more than an hour (something highly unusual for therapy patients). When the girl walked into his office smiling because she had peed every night, believing that he really didn't want her to, all the therapist did was smile, said, "Great, let's improve it," and took out a prescription pad. He wrote down "Drink 16 oz. of water before you go to bed every night; sleep home every night; and pee in your bed every night," and gave it to her. The third week the family came back for the appointment and the therapist kept them waiting over an hour and a half this time. He saw the girl for exactly two minutes, at which time he smiled at her response that she had peed in the bed every night, took out a pad, wrote down, "Drink 20 oz. of water every night before you go to bed; sleep home every night; and pee in your bed." By this time, the girl came to believe that this really was what the therapist wanted and by this point (keeping her waiting all this time after long drives and making her sleep home every night during the summer), he had become a much more obnoxious figure than her mother. She had no choice but to not pee in her bed because she certainly didn't want to cooperate with this "son of a gun." This case has been followed up for close to a year and the girl has not urinated in her bed one time since that fourth session.

A particularly effective but overbearing nurse who often irritated patients worked in conjunction with a doctor in a very successful way. The patient was a young man recuperating from a motorcycle accident. Because of his clinical depression, he would not motivate himself to go to physical therapy and do the kind of things he needed to do in order to be discharged from the hospital. The doctor saw that this nurse, who was the head nurse on his unit, particularly seemed to get under the patient's skin. He instructed the nurse at appropriate times to go in and talk to the young man and express her opinion that he probably shouldn't try to go to therapy yet because it was probably too soon for him. And in fact, she later made the messages even stronger by saying that she was sure he couldn't even do it yet, so he shouldn't push himself and shouldn't worry about that old doctor. Needless to say, the man hadn't lost his integrity so much that he was going to sit there and let this intrusive person act like an overprotective mother and tell him that he shouldn't, and even couldn't change. This became the motivation for the hard work that he needed to do.

THERAPEUTIC DOUBLE BINDS

In the old definition of the pathological double bind the victim is in a position where he or she can do not right. The classic example would be a double binding mother who comes home from work to her child and the babysitter, and when the child runs up to her and greets her, she responds to the child by saying, "Can't I have a few minutes' breather to myself when I first come home after a hard day's work?" And yet, when the child does not run up and greet her, his mother would say, "What's the matter? Working all day for you and I can't even get a greeting?" In this situation it becomes clear that the child is damned if he does and damned if he doesn't. In the therapeutic double bind, health professionals put themselves in a position where neither they nor can the patient can lose. The patient is changed if he does something and changed if he doesn't.

A social worker was running an assertiveness training group for women at a local mental health agency. One woman complained that, given her upbringing, it was impossible for her to say no to anybody with a legitimate request. The social worker gave her an assignment for the following week that she was to say no to at least three different people. The double bind, of course, was that the woman would either have to say no to three people, trying out a new behavior that probably would be helpful to her, or she would have to say to the social worker, "No, I won't do that assignment." Either way, the woman is forced into the position of saying no, which is what she claims she can't do. The subsequent learning is likely to be healthy for her.

EMBEDDED COMMANDS

Embedded commands are being mentioned here as well as in the next chapter on metaphorical communication. The process involves inserting one message aimed at a person's unconscious in the middle of a general sentence directed toward the person's conscious mind. The unconscious message is marked by a subtle tonal shift, a pause, a gesture of the hand, or a momentary eye contact, to mention just a few of the possibilities. By using these embedded messages, you can take a small fragment of a longer communication and allow that fragment to stand out in the person's unconscious as the critical message.

A physical therapist tells many of her patients messages similar to this one: "Most of the patients who DO THE EXERCISES like they're instructed to, come back and tell me that they START TO FEEL BETTER WITHIN JUST A COUPLE OF DAYS. I really enjoy when they return and tell me that." As the therapist speaks the words written in capitals, she subtly emphasizes them, either with a slight pause or with momentary eye contact or by talking slightly louder. While the person's conscious mind gets the general message that people improve when they do their exercises, the unconscious mind is getting the much more specific messages offered. The latter can potentially have a much greater effect on the individual's behavior.

It must be stressed that the presentation is not effective when kept at conscious awareness. If you obviously mark out the embedded message with very exaggerated tonality and/or amplitude, the person will realize what you're doing. In the examples we have presented, there would certainly be no harm in this, and it would probably even be somewhat effective. However, when done subtly and thus directed at the patient's unconscious, the effect is that much more powerful, mainly because there is no resistance to what is being said. If one consciously hears, "Do your exercises!" it can follow in that person's mind, "Well, I don't know if I'll really do it all" or "I'll do it maybe every other day," for example. When the unconscious hears it, it simply "sinks in" without any self-discussion. Of course, we are not saying that every embedded command will be followed directly, but that they have a high degree of effectiveness. It's often also a good idea to repeat the embedded message several times in different sentences. You make them that much more powerful.

"A long time ago when you were younger and smaller, there were a lot of things for you to learn that seemed difficult, even insurmountable, at the time. For example, remember when you were about a year old, give or take a month or two, and for the very first time you pulled yourself up against a chair, a desk, a sofa, somebody's hand, and stood up and put one foot in front of the other and started to walk. I'm sure you fell right back down again, and then got up again, and then fell back down again. But then eventually you learned to—(pause) *stand on your own two feet, Michael*—(pause) and that must have made you feel good." That is an example of what we call early learning sets. It's important for health professionals, whatever their particular profession happens to be, to remember that everyone has a history of doing things—such as learning to walk, talk, ride bikes, say the alphabet, read, and write—that at one time seemed so difficult, so impossible. They thought they could never do it, but now it is so everyday and ordinary that they can't even remember when it was difficult. In casual conversation it is important to remind people of that, since most of the time they're coming to a health professional because of something that seems out of their control. So within this generally healthy therapeutic message, which can be delivered in casual conversation anyway, there is one part that says, "stand on your own two feet" and then the patient's name, which can be embedded in there through pauses, as indicated above, and with a slight raising of the tone of the voice so that it actually becomes a separate command. If done well, this will not be noticed by the consciousness of the person, but the unconscious can pick it up and respond to it. More examples of embedded commands will be given in Chapter 7.

We know of health professionals who employ embedded commands in written material they give to patients. Such materials might include directions for taking medicine, for exercising, or for a diet. A subtly increased pressure of the pen for strategic phrases or sentences can help the patient's unconscious to receive their communications. For example, you may write "When you do these exercises, wear comfortable clothes" and push down more on your pen for the command "DO THESE EXERCISES." The mass media uses embedded commands on suggestions frequently by changing the type or using bolder printing for strategic messages.

CONFUSION TECHNIQUES

As each of you already knows, confusion is a very uncomfortable psychological state to be in. What you may not know is that each of you, and everyone else we know, has a tendency when confused to jump at the first logical suggestion you hear as a way of getting out of the confusion. Therefore, every effective health professional should have a variety of methods at his or her disposal and use creativity to dream up new ones when an old one is not appropriate, in order to utterly confuse the people around them. Of course after the confusion, one also needs to know how and when to slip in the appropriate directives to the patient. Below are a few examples that may help to confuse you even more about this topic.

A dentist had a young adult woman come into the office whom he had been seeing for about a year and whom he knew was particularly anxious around dental procedures. In her nervousness, she was making small talk as she sat in the chair and mentioned that she had just come back from an enjoyable vacation. The dentist told her that just before she came he had gotten a call from a friend who just came back from a vacation also. The dentist said that the friend was in the mood to . . . go to another state (this is, of course, a metaphorically embedded command for changing one's state from tense to relaxed) and that he lived near the border of the other state but didn't quite know how to get there. When he asked directions, the person in the gas station told him that he had to take two left turns and three right turns but neglected to tell him in what order. So the dentist's friend first took a right, a left, two rights, and another left, and he found out that that wasn't right. So in order to go back to where he had started from he then had to do the reverse so he made a right, two lefts, a right, and a left, and then he was right back from where he left. And he decided that this time he'd try it a different way so this time he made a left, three rights, then another left, and he found out that wasn't right either. So again he had to go back to where he left from by making a right, three lefts, and a right, and then he was right back there again and he thought, "How can I get to where I want to go?" He said to himself, "Well, I think I'll try it this way. This time I think I'll maybe start with two rights and then do two lefts and then do another right." And he looked around he saw that wasn't right either. So he thought, "Well, I'll have to go back to where I started." Whereupon he made a left, two rights, and two lefts, and then he was right back to where he originally left. And then he thought that he finally knew how to get to that other state. The dentist then said to the patient, "Now close your eyes and relax your jaw while I do this work." and the patient immediately followed that directive because it was a lot easier than to continue listening to that story.

One great confusion technique is to interrupt a motor skill that is habitual. For example, it is common for most people in our culture (particularly for men) to greet people with handshakes. Once one's hand leaves the body and starts out towards the other hand, the routine is almost automatic and an interruption of this causes great confusion. A particularly skilled male social worker we know will, when greeting a couple coming in for the first time for marriage counseling, stand up, walk across the room, extend his hand towards the man and when he reaches the man he will use his left hand to put the man's extended right hand in the air, which will confuse everyone greatly. He'll then say to the man, "Look at your wife and tell me all the ways she stabbed you in the back." He more often than not will get more intake data in the next two minutes, before the couple even sits down in the chairs, than he would have in a half hour of questioning using the normal routine. Again, he also starts off with certain assumptions. That is, if a couple is going to marriage counseling, then in some way or another they metaphorically feel that each is being stabbed in the back by the other.

There is a helpful technique for nurses on pediatric wards to use when going in to give oral medicine to patients who may not like its taste. Walk up, put the tray down, and then excitedly pantomime catching a fly or licking an ice cream cone. You will have fixed the person's attention and confused them so greatly as to exactly what you're doing that when you then offer the medicine, which is a logical nonverbal directive, the person will almost immediately drink it up. One of the authors remembers an experience when he was a teenager and in the hospital for surgery. He asked for a laxative, thinking it would be given in a pill form. That night the nurse walked in with a milk of magnesia and the author said, "There ain't no way I'm going to take that," at which time the nurse just broke out crying. This was so unexpected and confusing that the author just grabbed the milk of magnesia and gulped it down. The nurse apologized and said she was crying about a fight with her boyfriend. She then borrowed a dime to make a phone call, which the author gladly gave her just to get her out of the room. Again, the confusion was the discrepancy between the expectation of what the role of the nurse should be and her actual behavior.

As mentioned earlier in this chapter, one of the biggest drawbacks of these methods for health professionals is the belief that many of you must have after reading this—that these techniques are so silly and so obvious that the patient will obviously see through them and know what's going on and that there's no way these are really unconscious techniques. All we can tell you is that all three of us have used them many times and taught them to many students who reported back a voluminous amount of data to us. We know that more often than not the clients do not know what's going on and that this does effectively change their behavior without necessarily impinging on their consciousness. Once again, all we can do is suggest to you that you be adventurous enough to try something different and see, hear, or feel for yourself, what the outcome may be. You may be very curious to find out what changes happen with your patients.

EXERCISES

1. Identify the specific indirect communication technique that is illustrated by each of the following:
   a. Do you want to study for another one, two, or three hours?
   b. Since you're doing this exercise, you may as well start using these communication techniques.
   c. Actually, you probably don't have the courage to start using these techniques.
2. Pair up and, having one person play client and the other play health professional, from both positions give the other person in the dyad an incongruent message. Discuss. Switch positions and repeat.
3. What type of support would it take for you to begin to have the courage to use these techniques? Discuss as a class or in small groups.

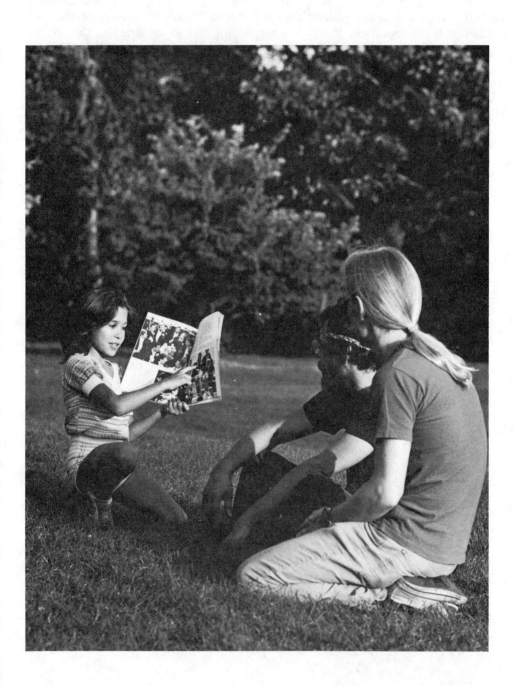

Metaphors—The Art of 7 Storytelling

Throughout the ages, the use of metaphorical stories, tales, fables, and anecdotes has been widespread and quite common. Philosophers, wise men, and storytellers have used such tales to teach, socialize, and help people to learn and resolve life's dilemmas. It is the belief of the authors that telling stories is the most elegant way to communicate. Added benefits are that the use of storytelling provides the communicator with the opportunity to be creative and, in suitable instances, to have fun.

Generally, a metaphor may be described as communication in which one thing is described or expressed in terms of another. As a result, some new light is shed or some new learning takes place in reference to that which is being described. Milton Erickson was a master in the use of metaphor. Only on rare occasions in therapy did Erickson speak directly to a subject or about a therapeutic problem with which someone was confronted. All of us grew up hearing fairy tales, stories, and anecdotes. Health professionals will find that the use of storytelling will, in almost all cases, be readily accepted by the person to whom the story is being told.

Like the other indirect communication forms discussed in Chapter 6, telling stories is an effective means of bypassing conscious resistance and communicating directly to the patient's unconscious resources for therapeutic change and problem resolution. It may be assumed that the more indirect and hidden a metaphor is, the more effective it will be in avoiding a patient's conscious resistance to change. However, the authors have found that even when it is obvious that parallels to a patient's life are being made in a metaphor, significant change can take place.

CREATING THERAPEUTIC METAPHORS

You may ask—"How do I create stories?" One way to start is to realize that you already regularly tell stories and use metaphorical statements in order to illustrate a point. Some may not be as subtle as you may deem necessary for the very clever patient, but sometimes the situation doesn't call for anything

91

profound. For instance, children are excellent candidates to relate metaphors to. You may want to begin your storytelling in such nonthreatening situations.

In creating a story for your patient, many of the forms of creative communication previously discussed in this book should be kept in mind. Most importantly, the story should *pace* the patient's world at least to some degree. Therefore, the hero of your story should use the same primary *representational system* (visual, auditory, or kinesthetic) that is used by your patient. Listen and make note of the words, especially the verbs, that your patient uses in discussing the situation and embed these words in your story. Quite often, a patient will use symbolic *organ language* in describing symptoms. which illustrates how he or she has unconsciously somatized stress. For example, a patient with migraine headaches may spontaneously use the expression, "what a headache he is!" A patient with chronic lower back pain may spontaneously remark that his job is "a pain in the ass."

Most importantly, a story should parallel in *structure*, but not necessarily in *content*, the situation related to a patient's symptoms or problems. Most often, this will involve the basic relationships taking place between the patient and other significant people or situations in his or her life. For example, a father with symptoms related to stress from family problems due to rebellious teenagers could be told a story about the captain of a ship dealing with mutinous sailors. Creative forms of communication such as *embedded suggestions* may also be included in the therapeutic metaphors that you tell your patients. Strategies such as *reframing* may be employed through the use of metaphor. Examples of therapeutic metaphors using some of these forms of creative and indirect communication will be presented in this chapter.

There are two main categories of therapeutic metaphors: (1) metaphors that provide a solution or several possible solutions to the patient's problem and (2) metaphors that access the patient's own unconscious resources for therapeutic change. In the latter category, there will be a signal or *accessing cue* in the story to symbolize the patient's unconscious resources. For example, the hero of such a story might have an encounter with a wise old magician who tells the hero a secret that provides the solution to his dilemma. Or the hero may meet with a Master Engineer who opens up an old dusty book to a particular page that shows a diagram illustrating how to build a bridge to get to the other side of the mountain. Or perhaps the hero will find a door that leads down into a basement that contains exactly the right tools he needs. Sometimes a therapeutic metaphor can provide a particular solution to a patient's problems *as well as* access the patient's own unconscious resources for resolution.

CASE STUDIES

In the following pages, numerous examples of therapeutic metaphors for a variety of clinical situations will be presented. As you read each example, be aware of how the story illustrates various characteristics of creative communication previously described in this book. It is of particular importance that the metaphor *pace* the patient. Italics will be used to indicate when a particular word or phrase is pacing the patient's language usage. Bold letters will be used to point out *embedded suggestions*. In many cases, the communicator would subtly emphasize such words or phrases with a tonal shift of the voice.

Case A

One of our students, Mrs. Thomas, was a nurse in a junior high school. She had a reputation for being a particularly effective communicator and nurse. As such, many of the students confided in her about their problems and looked to her for help. After school ended one afternoon, Mrs. Thomas was visited by a 12-year-old seventh grader named Richard. As they talked, the student proceeded to tell Mrs. Thomas of a bedwetting problem that he had that was, of course, quite embarrassing for him. Mrs. Thomas asked him how things were for him at home, and he stated that his parents often "pissed him off" and that sometimes he "felt flooded" with anger. He also stated that a brother and sister made him quite angry also. Mrs. Thomas learned that one activity that Richard particularly enjoyed was camping, and she proceeded to tell him the following story:

"You know, Richard, I love to go camping also. Last summer I went up to southwestern Pennsylvania to go camping along the banks of the Youghiogheny River. I hiked about ten miles upstream from where people go picnicking and rafting on the river to a town called Confluence, where there's a dam called the Youghiogheny Dam. Behind the dam is a large reservoir of water and there is a dam engineer who controls the locks of the dam allowing the water to flow through the dam and down into the river. I met the dam engineer, who told me that earlier that summer he had been having quite a problem. He said that two park rangers were particularly *pissing him off*. He also told me that campers and rafters downstream were making him angry. He said that in order to get back at these people, he opened up the locks of the dam and allowed too much water to pass through. As a result, the river was much too rough for people to have fun, and the job of the park rangers was also made more difficult. The dam engineer told me that when he did this, the rangers and the people in the park got angry at him, which got him even angrier, and he opened up the locks of the dam even more often. He told me that finally things were really getting out of hand and he wanted to close the locks of the dam, but it seemed like he had forgotten how. He was feeling quite distressed about his situation, but then he heard that the Master Engineer who originally built the dam was living in a cabin deep in the woods. The engineer went off to find the Master Engineer and after a long hike finally reached his cabin. He was invited in and behind the desk sat an old wise man with a long beard. The engineer told him of his dilemma and the Master Engineer reached behind him and brought out an old dusty book and placed it on the desk. He turned to a particular page and showed the dam engineer a diagram of exactly how the locks of the dam worked and then explained it to the engineer. They spoke for a few more minutes and then the Master Engineer said good-bye to the dam engineer, who left. When he returned, the dam engineer recalled what he had seen in the book and what the Master Engineer had said and found that he could **work the locks of the dam again, Richard**. He now knew how to work the locks so that he could **let just the right amount of water through** to the river. As a result, the people in the park and the park rangers were happy and this made the dam engineer happy. So Richard, I just wanted to tell you that story." At that point, Mrs. Thomas proceeded to talk about some other things with Richard. Several weeks later, she noticed him in the school hallway and asked how things were going for him, and was pleased to learn that his bedwetting had significantly decreased and that he was getting along much better with his family.

This therapeutic metaphor illustrates an example of utilizing the patient's own unconscious resources for problem resolution. It is also interesting to note that there really is a Youghiogheny River and a reservoir ten miles upstream in the town of Confluence. The nurse had been camping near the river several years ago and utilized the surroundings to create this metaphor.

Case B

Mr. Smith, a successful physical therapist, often uses metaphorical communication with significant effectiveness. Recently he was completing the last of a series of physical therapy sessions with a middle-aged male patient named Tom, who had been suffering from a degenerative disc of the cervical spine. Over the course of their sessions together, Mr. Smith learned that his patient was the oldest in a large family and that the patient had always "shouldered most of the burden" as far as family problems were concerned. This had continued to the current time, when the patient was "carrying most of the weight" for the responsibility of caring for his elderly parents. Mr. Smith also learned that his patient had been a Korean War veteran and highly decorated for heroic behavior for which the patient felt quite proud. Mr. Smith shared with the patient stories of his own military service. He spoke at length about how his platoon had won several awards for team work and how they accomplished some very challenging objectives by learning to **divide responsibilities, Tom**, and equally divided the weight of the duties assigned to them. When Mr. Smith saw Tom for a follow-up visit several months later, he was pleased to learn that the patient had asked his brothers and sisters to share the responsibilities and burdens of caring for their parents. Mr. Smith was also quite pleased to learn that the patient's neck pain was greatly improved.

Case C

Both metaphors presented thus far have both utilized *persons* as the main category of experience. It is important to know that any category may be used in therapeutic metaphors. Quite often, the health professional will want to use a category of experience that best paces the patient. For example, Dr. Jacobson was recently treating a female patient who had sustained considerable tooth damage due to bruxism. This condition, which involves a gnawing of the teeth, usually at night while the patient is sleeping, is most often caused by unexpressed anger. In speaking with his patient, Dr. Jacobson learned that she was an avid horse lover. Dr. Jacobson also was able to learn from his patient that she felt considerable frustration and anger because she was *only a housewife* and often felt shut in at home. The patient admitted that she had the freedom to get out of the house and do other things. However, she felt obligated to perform duties at home and often felt guilty if she behaved otherwise. The following week, when his patient was there for an office visit, Dr. Jacobson proceeded to tell her of a horse he owned years ago. The horse caused quite a problem and was an expense because the mare was always chewing through bits and harnesses that were placed around her mouth. He said that when the horse was finally allowed to roam out of her corral and graze in the fields, the equipment that was used lasted much longer. Dr. Jacobson added that the horse always returned back to the corral and to her stall at the end of the day. The patient returned two weeks later saying that she had told her husband that she wanted to get out and join a local tennis club. Her bruxism had significantly subsided as well.

Case D

Several years ago, one of the authors was visited by a male patient who complained of sexual dysfunctions of impotence and premature ejaculation. In gathering data from the patient, it was learned that his occupation was a plumber. The patient also stated that he had been married for a number of years, but that his wife became disenchanted with the relationship and, much to his surprise, chose to end the marriage about a year before. The patient stated that he soon began dating various women and experienced sexual problems with them. He stated that several weeks earlier, he met a "beautiful new woman named Pat" and was having the same problems with her. As a result, he decided to come in for treatment. This patient described his sexual problems with commonly used slang words and expressions. When the patient came in for his psychotherapeutic session the following week, the author proceeded to relate the following story:

"You know, you're a plumber, and I have a good friend who's a plumber. Several years ago, my friend had a contract to do all the plumbing work in a building. He thought he was doing a good job, but suddenly he was shocked when the manager of the building decided to terminate the contract. My friend went out to find another job and finally landed a contract to do all of the plumbing work in a beautiful new building. He went to work the first day but got numerous complaints from the tenants in the building. Some of them complained that there wasn't enough pressure in the pipes and the water didn't *come* out when they desired. Other tenants complained that there was too much pressure in the pipes and the water *came* out before they were ready. My friend left work that day feeling very sad and, on the way home, ran into a Master Plumber that he was acquainted with. They sat down and he told the Master Plumber what had been happening and the Master Plumber proceeded to tell my friend the following story." (This story on top of a story is what we might call a meta-metaphor.)

" 'I have a friend that I've known for many years who has always loved to play baseball. As long as I have known this fellow, he was always having fun playing ball. He played for his high school team and he had a lot of fun. When he graduated, a dream came true for him: He was drafted by the major leagues. He had a reputation for being a pretty good ballplayer and many people had great expectations of him. The day approached for his first big game and my friend, having been influenced by the expectations of so many others, decided that he was going to hit some home runs. Well, he struck out every time he was up at bat that day, and he made errors in his fielding. He was sitting in the locker room feeling very sad when Sparky, the experienced manager, came over to talk to him. Sparky told my friend that playing ball had always been a lot of fun for him but that he had gone out there that day trying to live up to all of the expectations that other people had had of him and that he had started to have of himself. Sparky told my friend to go out there the next day and to **just have fun playing ball** like he always used to. The next day, my friend went out on the field and the time came for him to *come* up to bat. He stood *firm* and *erect* at the plate, the ball came down toward him, and he *banged the hell out of it* and got a hit. He got a few other hits that day, did well in the field, and he went on to be a really good ballplayer.' The Master Plumber finished telling my friend that story, and then he leaned over and whispered a secret in his ear and told him that secret would be of great help to him in his plumbing work. The next day my friend went to work and everything went well for him. The tenants told him that there was just enough pressure in the pipes and the water *came* out only when they wanted it to. He had everything down *pat*." That patient went home and called the author several days later thanking him for trying to help him with his problems. He stated that somehow everything had worked out for him and he no longer needed any help.

This therapeutic metaphor is a good example of providing a solution to problems a patient is having (to have fun and stop trying to perform). It also illustrates an example of accessing the patient's own unconscious resources for the problem solving (when the Master Plumber whispered a secret into the plumber's ear). This metaphor also nicely illustrates how the strategic use of language can be used to pace the patient's situation.

Case E

Ms. Warren, a clinical social worker, was visited by a patient suffering from psoriasis. The patient, a young male, stated that he had visited several physicians and clinics that were not able to successfully treat his dermatological condition. The patient was open to the possibility that his psoriasis was psychosomatic and, therefore, sought psychotherapeutic treatment from Ms. Warren. In taking the patient's history, Ms. Warren perceived him to be quite angry under a facade of passive gentleness. The patient stated with a smile on his face that other people, especially his close family, often "got under his skin." At their therapy session the following week, Ms. Warren mentioned an artist friend of hers who had a reputation for painting beautiful pictures. However, recently his pictures had gotten progressively less pleasing to the eye, as the canvas began to be smudged up with irregular forms. The artist was quite distressed about this. He sat down to reflect upon what was happening to his artistic abilities and became aware that he had been getting upset with close colleagues and that they were *getting under his skin*. He became aware that he was taking out his anger on the canvas and decided that instead, he would begin to **safely and comfortably assert himself with his associates** and **let them know what he was feeling**. When he began to do that, his pictures became beautiful again. At their therapy session the following week, Ms. Warren's patient mentioned quite happily that his chest had started to become much more clear and healed of psoriasis. Several minutes later, he also mentioned in passing that he had been asserting himself more with people and "getting a lot of things off my chest."

Case F

One of the authors, a psychologist, was recently treating an adolescent for numerous behavioral problems. The teenager's parents were divorced, and the patient's father consistently called the author whenever the patient showed significant evidence of improvement. At such times, the father would point out things that were still wrong with his son. Clearly, the father had the need to continue to pathologize his son. Finally, when the son was much better behaviorally, the father asked for a conference with the author to point out things that were still wrong. On the afternoon of the father's appointment, the author arranged to leave his office door open so that the father in the waiting room could hear a call the author was making to a colleague. In actuality, the author called the weather on the phone, but proceeded to verbalize the following into the receiver:

"Yes, John, that wound could have been completely healed a long time ago. However, the parents have been very anxious and keep pulling the bandage off of her skin. When they do, it pulls the scab off and is interfering with the healing that can naturally be taking place. All right, I have to get off. I have a patient waiting."

At that point, the author invited the father in to hear the father's numerous complaints. However, the author had already communicated the message that was important to the father. This illustrates not only the use of metaphor, but also the use of an indirect means of delivering a powerful message.

Case G

A current health problem that many health professionals are consulted about is cigarette smoking. The authors have a colleague who is a nurse-practitioner and is very successful in helping people to stop smoking. She relies very heavily upon the use of metaphor and other forms of creative communication in her work, as the following case study indicates. She was recently monitoring the medication and treatment progress of a middle-aged woman suffering from high blood pressure. The patient, whose name was June, smoked two packages of cigarettes daily. She reported that she had tried to quit unsuccessfully on several occasions. She also reported that she began smoking as a teenager and that over the years both her parents as well as her husband and children had "been bugging" her to quit. The patient mentioned that cigarettes were "just like an old friend" to her. Over the course of several office visits, the nurse-practitioner managed to work into the conversation the following metaphorical communication: "You know, June, I can remember when I was working on my master's degree in nursing. I had finished all of the course work that was necessary, and all that was left for me to do was my thesis. For some reason it was taking me a long time to complete that thesis, and that was quite a problem for me. Every time I went home to visit my family they would ask me how I was doing on my thesis; they were always *bugging* me about it." The nurse-practitioner closely watched her patient's nonverbal cues for "yes" and "no" (see Chapter 4) as she continued to talk. "I don't know why I couldn't get that damn work done. Maybe I was angry at my family for bugging me and I was expressing my independence as a person by not giving in; maybe I liked the attention I was getting from them in some way; or maybe I was just lazy and didn't want to do the work." The nurse noticed that her patient emitted unconscious cues for "yes" at the suggestion that "independence" was the payoff for not getting the work done and that she communicated "no" signals for the other possible alternative payoffs. The nurse continued with the story: "Well, finally, I decided that the whole ordeal was making me sick, and I sat down to think about it one day. I became aware that I just didn't want to give in to my family and that not working on my thesis was my way of being stubborn and independent. I decided that since I was reacting to them so much, I really wasn't being independent, and that I had to do what was the right thing for me. Soon after that, June, I did the work necessary to complete my thesis. I have to admit, however, that now and then I continue to do certain things that are reasonably safe and comfortable just to prove that I am an independent person." Through the use of this metaphor, the nurse was able to learn what secondary gain her patient was getting from smoking cigarettes and thus reframe her patient's experience.

The nurse-practitioner also mentioned to her some sadness she was feeling because she recently learned that an *old friend* was acting in ways that were unhealthy to her and so she decided not to be friendly with the person anymore. Once, when the topic of children came up, the nurse-practitioner mentioned how she had recently seen a child playing in the middle of the street whose mother ran over, picked her up, and brought her to the safety of the sidewalk. She mentioned how the child screamed and protested because she was having fun, but of course, the child was young and didn't know any better and had to rely on the good judgment of her mother to take care of her. This was metaphorical communication to June that her body was just like a small child also. It couldn't make the correct decisions about care. June had to take the responsibility to take care of her body.

Finally, the nurse-practitioner told June the following story: "A friend of mine, April, was feeling sad recently and she didn't understand why at first. She finally became aware that she was having a problem saying no to men who wanted to have sex with her. She had the freedom, the power, and the choice to say yes if she wanted to go to bed with a man or to say no if she chose not to. So she began to assert that choice and independence and say yes when she felt like it and to **say no, June**, when she didn't and she felt a lot happier after that." A short time later June reported to the nurse-practitioner that she had decided to stop smoking and had successfully done so and that she felt confident to be able to continue "to have the power to say no."

Case H

Another common health problem is that of patients who are overweight or obese. A physician friend of ours was recently consulted by a young woman who was very overweight and suffering from related health problems. She complained that she had had no intimate relationships with men because of her weight and was desperate to do something about it. The physician learned that the patient had put on weight soon after being sexually assaulted some years earlier. He sensed that she unconsciously was using the weight to avoid relationships with men and that she felt safer and protected by being fat. He told her the following story:* "You know, Miss Smith, I have seen a lot of people in my practice, but I remember one woman 20 years ago who had a strange problem. This lady loved to take walks in a beautiful forest near where she lived. But one day, as she was walking down the path, a rodent came out of the bushes and scared her quite a bit. She ran home and would not come outside again unless she wore many layers of clothes around her body. She wore several shirts and sweaters and several pairs of pants. She wore a hat and gloves and high boots and felt protected with all the clothing on her. Well, she looked ridiculous and was very uncomfortable walking around like that. One day she talked with an old and wise neighbor of hers and he gave her some advice. He told her to learn everything she could about all the animals in the forest—which ones were safe and which were dangerous. He told her to learn what to look for and what to listen for and, as she felt safer and safer, to take off a layer or two of clothing. She followed his advice and as she learned more about the animals and only as she felt more and more safe, she

---

*Thanks to Bandler and Grinder's workshop for the idea for this metaphor.

was able to **take off some of the unnecessary layers** of clothing she was wearing. Before not too long, she was wearing only what was suitable and appropriate when she went outside." This metaphorical communication took into account the payoff for being overweight and provided the patient with an alternative strategy.

METAPHORICAL DIRECTIVES

Another form of metaphorical communication is to give *metaphorical directives* (see Chapter 4 for a discussion of directives). Milton Erickson was famous for using this therapeutic strategy. He was once visited by a young couple having a sexual problem. The wife was dissatisfied with their sex life because she wanted more foreplay, whereas the husband was only interested in getting down to the "meat" of the matter. Erickson learned that both the husband and wife enjoyed cooking. The wife enjoyed cooking appetizers and desserts, whereas the husband was a "meat and potatoes" man. He told them to go home and for two weeks prepare meals together. He directed them to both plan and prepare the appetizers and main courses for the meals. When he spoke to the couple later, Erickson learned that they were both satisfied with their sex lives. He had treated then entirely by using this metaphorical directive! Health professionals, especially psychotherapists and counselors, are often consulted by patients desiring to "straighten out" or "make a new life" for themselves. Metaphorical directives to go home and "clean out the basement" during the week, "throw out old food from the refrigerator," or "redecorate" a room can be very therapeutic.

Most times when we do workshops and teach this material, students end up asking two very important questions. The first one is, "What are the patients going to think of our telling these ridiculous stories that have nothing to do with their treatment? Won't they understand that it's really directed toward them and doesn't it seem silly?" The answer is no! On the contrary, most patients seem to enjoy the stories. In all the years we've been doing it, none of us has ever had a patient verbalize their recognition that the communication is metaphorical and no one has ever complained that we're wasting time telling stories that don't relate to him or her. We believe that if you have paced your patient and if your intent is to truly be of help (which, of course, would be the case), then in some way your patient will sense this and be accepting of your communication. Again, all we suggest is that you try it for yourself. It's very important that in order to keep these metaphors unconscious you make the situation different enough from the patient's situation that he or she doesn't recognize it. In fact, if you're telling the story and you notice that the patient begins to see similarities between himself or herself and the hero of your story, you casually create a discrepancy by saying, for example, that this girl had blond hair and was five feet ten inches tall (as opposed to the patient)—or you can casually drift away to an entirely new subject. Another technique is to make the metaphor really seem true, so that the patient is totally absorbed and doesn't even think of any conscious analogy to himself or herself.

A second and perhaps more important question is how and when to deliver these metaphors and stories. The best way to do so is casually in what seems like a break or before a session starts or after it ends. It is very easy to do an indirect communication technique "before the session starts" because the patient has no defenses geared up at that time. As you are walking them into the office, or casually giving your medication in a hospital room, or during a physical therapy session—if you deliver these metaphors in a casual, small-talk manner, the patient will in no way be attuned to analyzing your stories or discussing them in any more detail. Yet they will clearly hear, see, and feel all the things what you need them to experience for the result you're after.

EXERCISES

1. Let one student in your class or seminar portray a problematic patient whom he or she is working with or knows of. The student should portray the patient as much as possible (with physical gestures, language, and symptoms) while the other students ask the patient questions in order to collect necessary data. After collecting data, break up into groups of four or five and, as a group, construct a therapeutic metaphor for the patient. Now, allow one representative from each group to tell the metaphor to the patient (one at a time, of course). Regroup, and discuss the experience.
2. List as many common and widely used metaphors or symbolic types of statements (e.g., "a heavy heart") as you can.

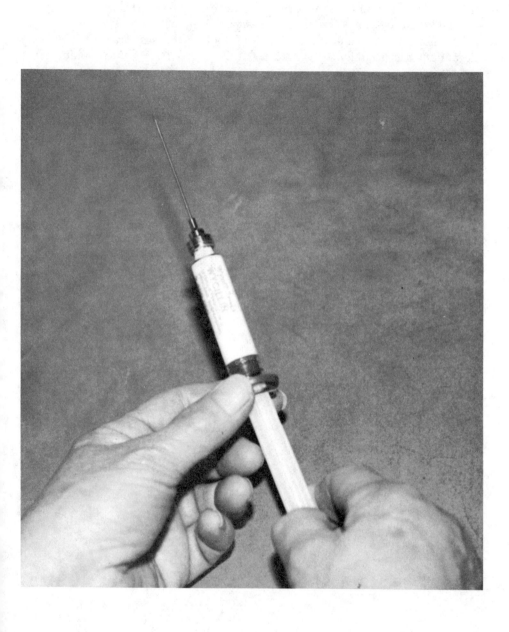

Anchoring 8

Kindly lean back in your seat and follow these instructions.

Remember a time within the last several years when you were involved in a really exciting situation. Vividly recall that time and as you do, actually step into the picture so that you can see everything around you as it originally appeared. Begin to be aware of the bodily feelings and sounds that accompanied that episode as you continue to remember the whole experience from start to finish. Allow yourself to CLOSE YOUR EYES, opening them only after you've completely gotten in touch with this experience, and please DO IT NOW.

Suppose that while you were absorbed in the previous experience, a specific stimulus, such as a sound or a touch on the shoulder, had occurred. If that same stimulus presented itself within the following several minutes, the same visual images and/or feelings from the initial experience would probably be elicited. We call this phenomenon *anchoring*, which will be the subject of this chapter.

This may, of course, sound like a familiar concept. It stems from the famous experiments of the Russian scientist Ivan Pavlov. He discovered that if you sounded a bell each time that you presented food to a dog, the dog would eventually begin to salivate in response to the bell alone. This process is referred to as classical conditioning. The same phenomenon occurs all around us and in our communication and can be used purposefully to allow the people you are talking with to have more choices in the way they see, feel, and hear.

By the use of anchoring, we can help make available to patients certain feeling states that would not otherwise be possible. This presupposes that we realize that each person already possesses all the resources he or she needs to face any situation. Sometimes, though, these resources are so far from conscious awareness that they cannot be utilized at a given moment.

For example, a patient may notice that each week just before he gets his allergy shot, he experiences a feeling of helplessness and breaks out in a cold sweat, trembles, and feels very anxious. He says that he can't seem to find the control that he would like to have in these situations. Viewed from the context in the preceding paragraph, we naturally realize that he already does possess this resource of the feeling of control in other areas of his life. If you ask him about his job, his hobbies, or his other interests, he will almost definitely be able to supply an example of one or more situations in which he really *does* feel in control. As this feeling surfaces, it can then be anchored to the present environment, as will be demonstrated in the following pages.

ANOTHER NAME FOR A FAMILIAR CONCEPT

Before we go into case examples, we must point out that anchoring is a naturally occurring phenomenon. Everyone reading this has had certain feelings elicited by the sight of something. That is because that particular sight is anchored to past experiences and the feelings associated with those experiences. Certainly, emotional states can be aroused in each of you when hearing certain sounds, be they as positive as the sound of surf hitting seaweed on your favorite beach or as negative as the sound of a siren. What health professionals do not take into account is that oftentimes a patient will respond to them based on established anchors. Think of how most of you feel when you go into a dentist's waiting room. Every sight and smell of the waiting room triggers feelings; for many patients, unpleasant ones. Many physicians unwittingly start off on "the wrong foot" with patients just by wearing their white coats or surgical greens. Again, the sight of such dress triggers associations and feelings that may not be helpful for treatment. This is especially true for children, who often start to cry as soon as a person in a white coat is seen. Many psycho-therapists wonder why their clients report being better outside of therapy yet seem depressed every time they are in the therapeutic situation. That is because the very sight of the office and even the person who was present when the client wasn't feeling good retriggers this bad feeling, even if outside of therapy the client has improved significantly. We actually know some psychotherapists who have two different offices or two different chairs, the first for patients to come and do their initial work (or "dump their load," as they call it) and the second for the process of getting better and working through some final solutions to their problems. What we are suggesting is that as health professionals you at least be aware of how your presence and some of the accoutrements of your office can automatically set off certain feelings in some patients. What you do with this information is up to you, but it can be helpful and different for each patient. However, you should never start off with the assumption that you are a neutral stimulus and that whatever reactions you get from patients are unique to them.

We will proceed with some examples, so that you can understand how you can use the techniques of anchoring as part of the treatment process.

Roy is a 22-year-old man who sustained a comminuted fracture of the left tibia and has been in traction and in a long leg cast for about six weeks. The physical therapist is working with him on muscle-strengthening exercises. Today Roy says he is sick of doing his exercises and that he wants to be left alone. The physical therapist could realize that the patient is understandably depressed and not bother him any more. While this is certainly acceptable and sometimes very appropriate, it might not be consistent with the goals they had set up concerning the size and strength of his leg needed for the upcoming removal of his cast. Instead of releasing him for the day, hoping that he would feel differently tomorrow, the therapist began to engage him in a seemingly unrelated conversation. She gradually drew up to an appropriate context by asking him if he could recall a time in the previous few years when he had felt really powerful and resourceful as a solid young man, a time when he felt he really had full control of the world around him. As she watched him, she observed a shift in his breathing, increased redness in his face, his chin moving forward and up, and a slight smile across his lips. She then knew he was accessing the requested experience. As this happened, she firmly touched him on the left shoulder for a few seconds. After a little more unrelated conversation, she then said, "Now I want you to realize that your cast will be coming off very soon and that you'll be walking out of here shortly afterwards." She then placed her hand back on his shoulder and began to notice the same bodily changes occurring as before, when he had accessed that powerful time in his life. As this happened, she continued: "And you know that if you expect to support your weight when the cast is removed, you'll have to take responsibility for getting your leg in shape. Why not at least start the exercises and stop if it's too difficult." She then withdrew her hand. He agreed to start the leg exercises without further discussion.

An explanation for why this works is that initially the physical therapist was attempting to motivate a person who had feelings of depression, fatigue, and hopelessness. It is very difficult to be motivated to do anything with these types of feelings. Indeed, some depressed patients never leave their beds in the morning because it requires too much effort. It is much easier to be motivated if there are concurrent positive feelings occurring internally. By anchoring these good feelings and then bringing them back at the appropriate time, Roy was able to make the choice of doing the exercise. Note that it was still Roy's decision and that he still could have selected not to do the leg raises. However, by accessing the positive feelings, he then had two choices and was more capable of choosing the one that he thought was best for him. The physical therapist helped Roy to access the positive feelings by associating a touch with the original remembered experience. She then used the touch to recreate the feelings at a therapeutically functional time.

The above example illustrates several salient points of effective anchoring. A touch of the body was used to establish the anchor and thus it can be referred to as kinesthetic anchoring. It is important that the anchor be of the same firmness and at the same location each time it is used. Touching the shoulder two inches away from where it was touched the first time or exerting different pressure the second time would not have elicited the same response as it did in our example. The timing of establishing the initial anchor is also crucial, though not difficult. As the physical therapist was asking the patient to recall a time when he felt powerful, she noticed changes begin to take place in his body. Only as these were becoming evident did she touch his left shoulder. This is very different from simply asking someone to recover some feelings and touching them just after asking, regardless of what they are experiencing at the moment. It is important that the anchor not be established until the communicator observes the desired nonverbal response, since the intention is for the touch to be associated with a specific feeling response and not simply the words asking for the response.

ACCESSING ANCHORS CONGRUENTLY

Again, as in all the other techniques as have discussed, congruence on your part is critical. This is another characteristic that is difficult to convey in the written word and was thus not evident in our initial example. When instructing someone to recall a particular experience, it must be asked for with the nonverbal language appropriate to that experience. When asking a person, for example, to remember a time when he or she felt really happy, the instructions must be delivered with the body movements and tonality suggesting a happy situation. The communicator must in essence move and talk like a person experiencing "happiness," when eliciting this from the person. Students have sometimes complained that they have had difficulty in getting a person to access a particular experience so that it can then be anchored. Lack of communicative congruence when eliciting responses is the major cause of this failure. Often exaggeration is needed, as long as it does not become obvious to the patient.

YOU'RE ALREADY DOING IT

Anchoring is another one of those phenomenon that we already use unconsciously in our behavior. Most of you can probably recall the time when you have gone up to a friend who was engaged in a particularly trying situation and firmly put your hand on his shoulder as you offered words of strength and support. At that time you had some sense that you had gotten the response you wanted. How did you know this? What made you "sense" this? You may now realize that perhaps it was the dropping and softening of the person's shoulders under your hand with maybe a slow, deep sigh accompanying it. When you later saw that same person, you instinctively placed your hand on the same shoulder with the same pressure and again had the sense of that same positive response. This and similar situations remind us of how commonly this phenomenon occurs around us. By allowing it to become part of your conscious repertoire, however, you can begin to use it in a positive, systematic manner. You can also begin to notice those times when, like most of us, you sometimes use anchoring with negative consequences. You can then learn to limit this type of pattern, as will be illustrated.

A physician on rounds walks into the room of an elderly patient with a long-standing pneumonia and situational depression. As the patient is telling the physician how sad and helpless everything seems, the physician takes the patient's hand in hers and says that she understands. Several days later she walks in and sees the patient sitting up comfortably in bed and talking to his neighbor. The nurse reports that he has been ambulating and seems 100 per cent improved. As the physician sits down at the bedside, she takes his hand in the same manner that she did previously. Within a few moments the patient's face turns to gloom as he again begins to complain about how bad he feels. The physician leaves frustrated, thinking that this is another one of those crabby old patients who likes to bitch and stay in the hospital as long as possible. Little does she know that she is unintentionally going around and actually helping to create these nasty old patients. Notice that this is entirely different from our example of going up to a friend and offering support and words of strength. In that case, strength and support were being anchored, as evidenced by the body's response to the shoulder touch. In the second example, feelings of depression are being anchored. The fact that the physician honestly intended support and understanding by her touch does not matter in this situation. To be fair, this hypothetical situation must be looked into a little further. If, when visiting the patient on the day he was feeling better, she had sat down on the bed presenting a cheerful face and a happy tonality to her voice at having heard the good news from the nurse, the result could definitely have been different. Even though the negative anchor of her hand touching the patient's hand would have been present, this probably would have been cancelled by the generally positive visual and auditory anchors of her facial expression and voice tonality. If, however, like most of us, she was busy thinking about the mechanics of her case (such as medications and pending lab tests), while visualizing her patient's most recent x-ray in her mind, her calculated voice and facial expression would probably been the same as they were the previous day. Thus, not only the feeling of her hand, but the look on her face and the sound of her voice would have served as three powerful anchors to access the patient's previous negative feelings. This example shows us how at any moment we are all being exposed to numerous anchors: visual, kinesthetic, auditory, and sometimes olfactory and gustatory. This also obviously means that if we can purposefully present people with anchors in more than one mode at a time, the feelings that we can elicit will be even that much more powerful.

TONAL ANCHORING

A type of anchoring that we use a great deal is tonal anchoring. This occurs when we shift the tone or tempo of our voice in association with a particular response. Thus it is the exact same idea as kinesthetic anchoring, except that we use the voice to establish the anchor.

Peter is telling Susan about a recent vacation he has taken. Every time he mentions "the beach" he slows down, softens his voice, and stretches out the word in a dreamy fashion. Each time Susan hears "the beach" her face reddens a bit and her breathing slows down, her mouth opens, and her shoulders drop down gently. The words, "the beach," spoken with a characteristic tone, pitch, and tempo have become an auditory anchor for these feelings of relaxation in

Susan. It must be stressed that, in the same way as with kinesthetic anchoring, the tonal and tempo shifts do not by themselves establish an adequate anchor—they must be initially paired to a definite response in the person to whom they are being offered. In our example, if Susan had either not been listening or had been thinking of a time when she walked on a beach when it was cold and rainy, the relaxation response would not have been elicited. Communicators need to observe clear sensory output to be aware of what response is going to be anchored, instead of what response they think should be occurring at a given moment.

Tonal anchoring is a phenomenon that is going on around us all the time. Think of how many times a member of your family has said something in a tone of voice that immediately aggravated you. In jargon this is referred to as "having your buttons pushed" in response to something someone says. Or we may say that someone is "making us upset" by the manner in which he or she is saying something. We hear something said in a particular manner and are automatically propelled into our characteristic way of feeling in response to the tonal anchor. This is another reason why we don't consider our forms of communication either manipulative or evasive—these phenomena already occur all around us. To use them responsibly with conscious awareness, keeping in mind desired outcomes for patients, instead of allowing them to occur haphazardly with varying or perhaps unwanted results, is, we believe, behavior that is entirely consistent with the service-oriented goals of health professionals.

VISUAL ANCHORING

Accessing feelings through a visual anchor is also very prevalent in human behavior. Think for a moment of all the things you see around you that by their sight alone evoke certain responses: a country scene, a certain magazine cover, a particular outfit on a friend or spouse, a certain facial gesture such as the raising of eyebrows—these are examples of visual anchors. What responses can you note in your body at the exact time when we ask you to imagine a white pony running in a beautiful green field or a woman wearing six-inch heels, a wig, red tights, and a matching handbag, sauntering straight toward you? While you're at it, you may begin to realize what a strong anchor the sight of a needle on a syringe is to a patient. Notice in the next 24 hours how many times you feel some emotion simply in response to seeing something or somebody. Visual anchors can also, of course, be used purposely in communication. Instead of associating certain touches or voice tones to certain responses, visual gestures or body movements can be offered. For instance, imagine you are in a clinical situation where you want to anchor feelings of confidence so that you can utilize them later, if you notice the patient becoming hopeless again. As you ask the patient to recall such an experience (when he or she felt REALLY confident) and then notice that the patient is doing so, you shift your shoulders and raise an eyebrow or place an extremity in some characteristic position in front of you. If done covertly and timed correctly, the same pose struck later will evoke the same feeling of confidence, which can be utilized therapeutically.

A well-known therapist and teacher of many of these patterns of communication, Judith Delozier, uses another type of visual anchoring in her practice. She usually keeps a vase of roses in her room. Near the beginning of a session she will have her client access some positive experience. As she notices the response, she uses the roses as an anchor by glancing over towards them herself, noticing that the client does the same. During the remainder of the session, when the client begins to slip into certain types of negative feelings, such as those of helplessness and inadequacy, she simply again looks toward the roses. The client looks also, and it becomes obvious from the dramatic bodily changes of the client that the roses have become a powerful anchor. With the positive feelings restored, changes can often be achieved more rapidly and effectively.

KINESTHETIC ANCHORING

Several other examples of primarily kinesthetic anchoring will now be presented. Kinesthetic anchoring is the easiest for most people to learn and therefore approriate to use when first attempting the technique. Also, kinesthetic anchoring is the most irresistible of the three types; even if a patient is not looking, listening, or concentrating, he will still be able to feel a touch somewhere on the body.

Example A

An occupational therapist, Susan, is working with a middle-aged woman who has rheumatoid arthritis, and is instructing her in exercises of fine motor coordination of the hands. As discussed at a recent interdepartmental team meeting, Martha usually stops working after a couple of minutes, complaining of a lack of stamina. This time she again says that she is too tired to continue, that her hands hurt, and that she would like to return to her room. Pacing her experience, Susan says that she notices how tired Martha looks; why don't they stop working for a while and simply sit down and chat. After some casual conversation, Susan asks Martha if she can remember a time in the near past when she was too tired to do something but somehow did it anyway. Martha replies, "No," that she can't ever do anything because she's always too tired. Noticing the unsuccessful outcome of this last communication, Susan modifies her own behavior and this time much more congruently says, "Surely there must have been some time in the last couple of years when a task seemed insurmountable, yet you realized that you were the only one who could manage it, and you did it successfully." As Martha's eyes shift up and right and then up and left, she sasys that indeed there had been a time one year ago when she had been feeling really weak, when her husband's sister and husband suddenly announced unexpectedly that they were visiting from out of town. She had no energy to spare, but liked these in-laws and didn't want to disappoint them or her husband. With some help from him she managed to be a good hostess and even enjoy the weekend. Martha smiles and while tilting her head and nodding she exclaims in a congruent tone that she really remembers being surprised that Sunday night at being able to do as much as she did with as little effort as it seemed.

As she related the story, Susan noticed the changes that were occurring in Martha's voice tone and body language. At that point, Susan placed her hand casually on Martha's midback and then exerted moderate pressure when Martha told her about how well she had done. After a little more conversation, Susan wanted to test her anchor to make sure it was firmly established. As they stood up, Susan asked Martha to come back that afternoon—that she was sure they could make real progress if tey really tried together. While saying this, she put her hand in the same position on Martha's back, exerting similar pressure. She immediately noticed the same smile, tilting of the head, and nodding as Martha said that she thought it was a definite possibility. When Martha returned that afternoon, Susan fired the anchor in a similar manner at the beginning of the session and several times during the remaining period whenever things would slow down. Although Martha never totally stopped complaining, she did so to a much lesser degree and satisfactorily completed all of her remaining sessions with Susan.

Example B

Another illustrative case involves a dental student, Alan, who had heard about anchoring and was anxious to try it. A woman entered his examining room one day and while sitting down casually remarked that she was going to be a "difficult one" because she was really afraid of injections. He made no specific reply to this and simply started to examine and x-ray her teeth. After it was apparent that she had several large cavities that would require local anesthesia, he sat back down next to her and started to re-examine her teeth. As he did this, be began talking about some experiences he had had recently. He led toward asking the patient if she could recall a time in the last few years when she had thought that something was going to be really difficult or scary, but that it turned out to be a breeze. To let her talk, he removed his instruments from her mouth but kept his arms close to her so that he could anchor her right shoulder with his left upper arm when it became appropriate. He did this because he knew he would not have a free hand when he would need to fire the anchor again. The patient remembered a recent vacation at the beach and how she had refused to go into the water because she thought it was too cold. Each day she told herself that she wanted to go in, but after feeling the water with her feet decided that it would be too painful. Finally one day she decided that she was not going to put up with her fear any longer. She simply took a deep breath and ran right in until she was completely submerged. To her surprise, the water had hardly seemed cold at all, and she completely enjoyed herself for half an hour. As she reached this part of the story, he anchored her in the manner described.

A few moments later while firing the anchor, he related his findings. He observed that even though she verbalized feelings of fear, she did not seem to get very upset. As he returned with the syringe and proceeded to inject, he again fired the anchor. She groaned several times, hunching up her shoulders, pushing him away once, and wiggling in her chair, all for about twenty seconds. However, she then settled down and let him administer the injection without further event. He told us later that as he was putting the needle away, he felt disappointed that the anchoring technique had not worked. However, as he was thinking this, the patient began saying how surprised she was that she behaved better with this shot than ever before. She usually got so worked up that it took at least five or ten minutes to get her to calm down enough in order to cooperate, and even then she would remain totally frightened.

These two examples may call to mind some of the potential situations in which you may be able to use anchoring successfully in your own work. Most health professionals share a particular advantage in doing kinesthetic anchoring because in the health field there is naturally a lot of body contact. Whereas other professionals might find it difficult to reach out and touch the person they are communicating with, we are often in a situation in which physical contact to the shoulder or back would not seem too invasive.

SELF–ANCHORING

A common question is whether people can fire their own anchors. The answer to this is yes. Note how common it is for someone to place one thumb on the temple and the second and third fingers on the other temple to access the state of concentration. People in many meditation disciplines will often begin by assuming a characteristic body position that enables them to enter their desired state that much easier. In the same way, patients can be taught to utilize anchors by themselves. One can anchor feelings of safety and support, for example, with a particular type of patient who feels very frightened and powerless to face his or her disease. The anchor could be a squeeze of that person's hand. Thereafter the person could be shown that that hand could be squeezed any time that feelings of safety and support were needed.

The same potential exists for visual anchors. People can use surrounding objects to evoke the desired experience. We all utilize this method when we wear a particular blouse or suit that helps us to feel good or confident. The health professional can also utilize objects to help patients with desired outcomes. For example, a neighborhood pharmacist was asked for help by a patient who tended to doze off at the wheel of her car. He instructed the patient to engage in eight sessions of vigorous exercise. Just before each session she was to put on a cap with a rim. After the exercise sessions she was told to put on the cap and drive (with another person at first, just to be safe). The cap provided both kinesthetic and visual (the rim of the cap) anchors for alertness, and the patient was able to drive safely.

BUT WILL THEY LAST?

A question often asked is how long these anchors last. The answer is, of course, that the length of time is extremely variable. If the original event was intense, then the anchor associated with it could last for decades. For many people, the sight of blood is anchored to some unpleasant experience that happened very early in life. The experience may be fear and/or helplessness. That anchor is often sustained throughout a lifetime. Other anchors may last only 30 minutes. The use of anchoring in the clinical setting is not dependent on the anchors lasting a long time. Anchors are useful simply in helping others achieve a new desired state of experience in a particular situation. Once they experience this new emotional state, the anchor is no longer needed. For example, the person who always exhibits symptoms of extreme anxiety before injections is asked to remember a time before an exam when he or she felt a little apprehensive, but very confident. These feelings are then anchored. If the anchor is fired just before the injection, the patient is able to get through it with a minimal amount of anxiety. The anchor is thus no longer necessary because the patient has had a direct experience of a relatively painless occurrence that will always be available to him or her.

COLLAPSING ANCHORS

Another application of anchoring is what Bandler and Grinder call "collapsing anchors." This technique is valuable when there are two or more experiences, behaviors, or attitudes that can be valuable to the patient and that you wish to "anchor in." Dr. James is treating an administrator for hypertension. The patient works very hard during the day, brings work home at night and on weekends, and rarely takes vacations. He admits that he knows how to relax but is reluctant to do so because "hard work has made me a success." Dr. James asks his patient to remember the last time he really felt relaxed and touches him on the left shoulder as the patient does so. A few moments later, Dr. James acknowledges that hard work can be very important and touches the patient's right shoulder as the patient responds affirmatively. Then, as he and his patient agree that *both* relaxation and hard work are important, Dr. James fires both anchors. As he does so, he acts as if he is putting his hands on the patient's shoulders in order to be friendly. This technique assumes that all behaviors of a patient are potentially valuable resources and collapsing the anchors integrates the behaviors into the person's experience.

In closing this chapter, an example of the utilization of visual anchoring will, we think, further demonstrate the power of this phenomenon. As we have already said, the effects of anchoring are constantly going on all around us, usually without our awareness of them. The following episode involving one of the authors is no exception; only after the fact did he realize what had occurred. On the last day of his Family Practice residency, he came to work in a red derby hat and a long-sleeved T-shirt that had a design of a shirt and sport jacket and bright red tie painted on it. Viewed from at least several feet away, it looked as if he were actually dressed up in a tie and jacket. While on rounds with his patients that morning, the experience was truly memorable. It seemed as if everyone had suddenly decided to heal themselves as a going away present. A terminal cancer patient who would lie there expressionless from day to day actually beamed and said hello when the author came to his bedside that day. A woman who had been complaining of severe pain in different areas of the chest, back, and abdomen every single day without exception over a three-week period actually sat up in bed laughing, saying that she had had no more pain in the last several hours. Only after finishing rounds did the author realize what had happened. Usually when he would be about to enter a room he would imagine who he was going to see and how that person would be that morning. For example, with the woman who constantly complained of pain, he might picture her in bed wrinkling her brow and complaining of severe pain. He would then start talking internally, complaining about the situation to himself, and begin to feel frustrated and impatient about the whole affair. When he finally arrived at the bedside, the picture of himself that he presented to the patient was consistent with these feelings that he was having. This picture, complete with downtrodden face, shifting eyes, white coat, and stethoscope, served as a perfect visual anchor for her of the previous feeling she had had on other mornings when she had seen him. Thus, on the last day when she saw him in the hall on rounds with other patients and then in her own room, none of these original feelings were elicited. She was finally able to speak from her true experience and tell him exactly how her body felt that morning. Had he had any more days left, he might have next tried walking into rooms backward or on his hands. At least he will from now on realize the effect of his facial expressions and attire and adjust them when necessary.

One other encouraging by-product of that day was that no patient complained either to the author or to the nurses of the authors actions or attire. He had thought that at least one or two people might have been annoyed or uncomfortable—which would have been at least closer to the truth than the opinion of some of his colleagues, who thought that most of the patients would be outraged. Again, the great demand for a certain type of professionalism that we think patients had has been found to be more a function of our own imagination. Having the rapport he had with the patients was enough for them to not only accept, but enjoy and benefit from the unconventional way that he behaved.

No, don't be UNprofessional. Simply be effective, which *is* professional.

EXERCISES

1. Practice anchoring with your partner. Kinesthetic anchoring is the easiest to start with. For instance, while the subject is talking about some happy experience, touch a shoulder. Note the exact facial features, voice tonality, and breathing rate. After a minute or two, try the anchor again and note the effect. Have a third person in the group observe and verify your findings.
2. Identify common anchors in your environment: things that give you a certain experience when you see, hear, feel, taste, or smell them.

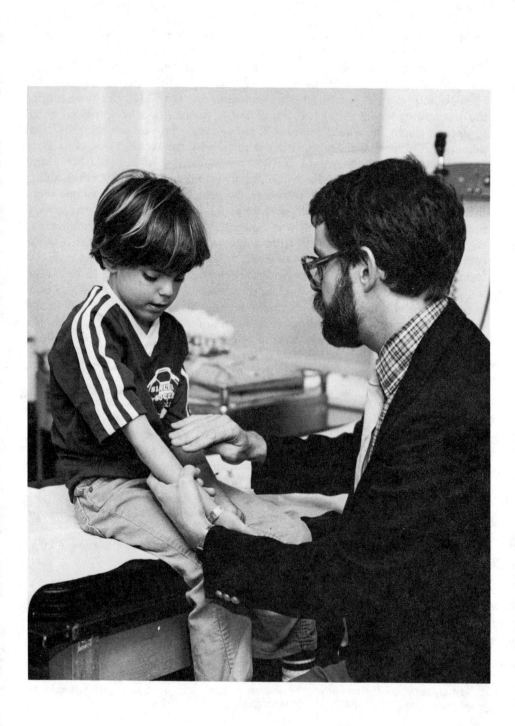

Relaxation and Attention–Focusing Techniques 9

Joseph Greenwald, the typesetting coordinator for this book, was not in very good spirits as he drove to his apartment from the West Coast office that evening. As he related to us several weeks later, they had just finished a particularly grueling day. He had wanted to finish work on the final chapter but instead was inundated with an unprecedented amount of calls and other matters of business that took priority. Even his lunch break had been hectic. He had had to run to the bank to get a certified check, so that he could catch a bus to the car dealer's to pick up his Datsun. All of this he would have settled for, but for the fact that the chapter had to be on his editor's desk by the next morning—at least three more hours of work were ahead of him. After stopping off to pick up some extra coffee and aspirin for the night he gloomily continued home. Walking into his apartment, he switched on the answering machine for messages. . . .

Frank, his typesetting partner, had called from the hospital. Although he had been experiencing a great deal of pain the day before, Frank's appendectomy wound was relatively pain free. His only trouble now was the prospect of having to lie there bored to death for two to three more days. Joe blankly stared at the tape machine as he heard Frank insisting that he would finish the final chapter, as originally planned, and had already arranged for a copy to be sent to him at the hospital that evening.

The first thing to come into focus were his keys as they still dangled from his hand. Slowly the rest of the room also came into view as he started to breathe more fully. Without wasting time, Joe ran down to his car and started a 15-minute drive to the beach. Smelling the water as he got out of the car, he laughed to himself as he suddenly realized that this time it didn't bother him in the least that he was getting sand in his shoes. As he watched the orange sun on the now almost deserted beach, he found a spot and plunked down.

He smiled and experienced great delight as he burrowed his hand into the sand and gently poured tiny grains over various areas of his suit. As he watched the sand sparkle against the sun, he realized that until that moment, the concept "don't get sand on your clothes," had been as real to him as "thou shalt not kill!" He saw that it was *he* that had created the "reality" that sand and "being dressed" do not mix. Actually, they went great together — as he started making little designs around his tie. He suddenly realized how he had similarly created the whole day gone wrong, resisting every event and calling them interruptions to his "real" work that he had wanted to get done. He realized that the day had actually been perfect, complete with calls, meetings, and appointments, and that the only thing that had turned it around was his constantly wanting it to be different. After experiencing some momentary sadness at this, he started to hear the sea gulls squawking and the breaking of the waves. Then, again, the smell of the ocean came in a rush and the perfect cool breeze played on his face and hair. He laid back and watched the setting sun, wriggling just a little deeper into the sand and feeling his muscles melting away. His body soon became so heavy that he wondered if he would be able to get up by the time the tide came up. Sand on his clothes was one breakthrough enough for the day—sea water was another story. He smiled and closed his eyes and drifted off for a while.

This chapter will be concerned with the various aspects and techniques of relaxation. One reason we include it in a book such as this is that often it is a necessary ingredient in the communication process. Although some of the techniques we have previously discussed can be used effectively with agitated patients, other strategies may call for a person initially being relaxed. People who are comfortable and relaxed are often much better equipped to follow instructions and suggestions, as will be illustrated in this chapter.

The second reason we address the subject of relaxation is that stress is directly related to many aspects of disease. Stress has been shown to lower normal immune mechanisms. Riley showed that by varying stress we could alter the incidence of breast cancer in mice from 92 per cent under stressful conditions to 7 per cent in a protected environment. He also discussed how the surveillance mechanism of the immune system is impaired by stress and how the decrease in this mechanism allows a more rapid growth of malignancy. Solomon and Amkraut showed that when compared with healthy children during a six-month period, those children who came from stressful environments were more susceptible to infectious diseases and had a longer recovery period.

Relaxation is also a medically accepted treatment for many disease states, such as headache, peptic ulcer, hypertension, and spastic colon. This chapter is intended to give the reader all the necessary information to successfully practice relaxation techniques in a clinical setting.

WHAT IS RELAXING?

What happens when we allow our bodies to relax? How is it that things that previously had a marked hold on us can suddenly be viewed in a completely different manner? Results of research in electroencephalogram (EEG) biofeedback, as well as certain disciplines such as Silva Mind Control, contend that when we relax completely, our brain enters an altered wave state that allows us to take in and assimilate information more expediently. Normal waking EEG patterns are usually in what is called the beta range, or a frequency greater than 14 cycles per second (c.p.s.). Normal sleep patterns fall below this. Delta, under 4 c.p.s., is considered deep sleep. Theta, or 4 to 7 c.p.s., occurs during normal sleep and alpha, 7 to 14 c.p.s., during dream sleep. The latter, or alpha level, falls just between the boundaries of normal sleep and normal wakefulness. It has been determined from numerous EEG experiments that many individuals can enter alpha levels while awake. Scientific literature has demonstrated that alpha brain wave activity is associated with tranquility, creativity, accelerated healing, concentration, learning, and ESP. It is possible, therefore, to view relaxation as such a shift in the mind's electrical activity.

Another more classical explanation of relaxation, and one that is not mutually exclusive of the former, sees it as primarily a muscular phenomenon. We are all keenly aware of the voluntary nature of the muscles of our arms, legs, eyes, and jaws. The muscles of our abdominal wall, back, neck, scalp, and chest are not as real to us in terms of assigned control. We "know" that they are voluntary, since we learned it in school and can do things like flex our abdominals to protect ourselves from a punch. However, we are not accustomed to controlling these muscles consciously. They certainly do contract, however, as we have all experienced in the progression of a typical day. What happens is that we gradually tighten them at an unconscious level. A red light, an unwelcome interruption, a threat, a negative thought, a disapproval—all of these things that occur a thousand times in a day are pushed somewhere into the muscular armor of our bodies. Some people have a predilection for storing this tension in their head and neck muscles; they are the ones who get tension and migraine headaches. Others put it in their abdomen and end up with such things as constipation, spastic colon, heartburn, and ulcers. Still others store it mostly in their back, with obvious results.

A few of you might find it hard to believe that simply tightening your muscles can cause real aches and pains. We urge you therefore to try this simple experiment, which can even be done as you continue to read. While sitting or standing, move your arm away from your body to a point where it is level with your shoulder. Simply leave it there for two full minutes. For your arm to stay in this anti-gravity position, the arm abductors—especially the deltoid muscle—must stay contracted. Probably even before the two minutes are up, you will start to feel first a heaviness or "tiredness," followed by actual pain. We've obviously all experienced this when we have used a particular muscle group for a greater than normal load or time span. Thus it should not be difficult to understand how continuous muscle contraction, probably through constriction of the fine blood vessels that run through the muscle's fibers, can lead to an experience of pain.

When we are tense, but not actually feeling a particular ache in the body, we instead experience a certain feeling state or emotion. Some examples are frustration, anxiety, tiredness, and impatience. One may be thinking, "All this work is really getting me upset, I can't wait to get out of here." Simultaneously, the person may be unconsciously experiencing a great amount of tension in the upper back and shoulders and neck. The problem is then multiplied by the fact that each successive event of the day is experienced and felt through these tensions and emotions. Thus, the way we view each person we encounter or each task we set out to do is colored and shaped by this filter. It is as if we were throwing pebbles into a large, smooth lake. It looks as if a pebble could have all the room it needs to laxily drift to the bottom. When we look closer, though, we see that the water is actually filled with dense mud, weeds, and other rocks, so that two inches into the water the pebble comes to an abrupt halt.

One begins to wonder how we can allow ourselves to be unaware of the tightness in our bodies. We could focus in on our bodies if we wanted to, just as the reader could focus now on the feeling of this book in his or her hand. The reason we usually don't, the authors believe, is that most of us have been socialized to learn that we have little control of our bodies. If we allowed ourselves to feel, for example, our tense abdominal muscles or lower back, we would be alarmed and not know what to do. When, however, we see it through a concept such as, "I feel lousy; I can't wait to get home," this gives us at least a momentary idea of some voluntary control. At the instant we picture ourselves resting at home, our body is experiencing a fleeting release, because we imagine that we will at least be able to relax at that time. Actually this is just an illusion of control, since the solution is always in the future instead of now. The idea of this chapter is to present techniques for helping patients learn to relax now instead of in an imaginary future. The relationship between relaxation or tension on the one hand and experienced pain on the other is clear. If you ever need to demonstrate this relationshhip to a patient, just take a dental probe, ask the patient to make a tight fist and stick the top of the hand with the probe. Then ask that patient to relax his hand and in the same spot with the same amount of pressure apply the dental probe. It is clear that the trial in which the fist was tight will be the one in which the most pain was experienced. We are not suggesting a direct psychological cause for all pain; but there's a prima facie case for the fact that tension alters the experience of pain. It should also be obvious that, except for a minimal amount of tension that can be a motivating factor, most tension is dysfunctional in terms of the patient's motivation to do what is needed to get better.

RELAXATION TECHNIQUES

The first technique is one with which you have all had direct experience—it was used in the story that began this chapter. This example includes many of the ideas already presented in this book and was in fact used exactly for this purpose. First, the story is a metaphor. We know of no such entity as a typesetting coordinator, and Joe Greenwald was created with a flick of our pens. As we suggested in Chapter 6, we purposely made him sound like a believable character to involve you more directly in the experience of the story. Note that "John Smith, an old friend of ours" might not have been as effective.

Another aspect of the story was that it probably adequately paced your experience. Though we are not assuming that all of our readers are tight knots of spastic muscular activity, we certainly remember our student years when at times there seemed to be too little time for too much work. Also, of course, many of the patients with whom we will be reacting will be in equally stressful situations. Since our idea in beginning the chapter was to give you a direct experience of relaxation rather than just talk about it, we realized that we first had to meet you at your level of the world as we imagined it before we could bring you anywhere else. Thus we started out with the eidetical story of our "typesetting coordinator." Once you were engaged, it was a much simpler task to lead you in the desired direction.

A third ingredient present here is indirect communication. When we read about "someone else's" experience, it is very difficult to resist getting into it ourselves. We didn't ask you to imagine yourself "snuggling even deeper into the sand," something that many of you might have resisted. While reading about Joe Greenwald, however, it is only natural that we float right along with him as he savors his experience. For those of you who did not take part fully in the exercise at the beginning of the anchoring chapter, you might notice whether this story was easier for you to get into.

This last remark brings to mind a fourth characteristic of the story, its use of a natural anchor such as the beach. For almost all of us, the word "beach" elicits feelings of comfort and relaxation. From the first mention of this word, these feelings started to set the stage for the remaining part of the story. (Of course, if you have a patient who has a phobia of water, you would not use a beach story to elicit relaxation.)

If you were telling the previous story directly to a patient, you would have had other tools to use that we did not have at our disposal. You could have started in a tone and tempo characteristic of the setting. You might have matched phrases to the patient's breathing and even breathed at the same pace yourself. As you progressed, of course, your voice could have gotten deeper and slower as you led the client deeper and deeper into the metaphorical sand. The point of this discussion is that the use of metaphor is one technique that is available to us as a powerful relaxation tool.

The Deep Muscle Relaxation Technique

The classical relaxation technique is actually not one set exercise but variations around a common idea. The essence of it is simply to consciously relax each muscle of the body in stages. It begins with having the patient sit in a relatively quiet area. We think of relaxation as an active process in that the subject must begin to do something that is different from his or her normal state of consciousness. A behavior that is often first chosen is slow and deep breathing.

A tense person breathes in a shallow and rapid manner, whereas someone who is feeling relaxed will usually be breathing in much the opposite manner. The breathing must be worked on during the entire procedure. Even though you say breathe slowly and deeply, the subject will often breathe at two to three times the desired rate. Accept (pace) that rate and then continue to slow it down. Do this both by directly telling him or her to slow down and by indicating this with your own body language, such as beginning to talk more slowly and deeply and in rhythm with the breathing.

When satisfied with the breathing, the next thing is to begin to have the patient focus in on specific anatomic muscle groups. We prefer beginning at the feet. One can tell the subject either to begin to feel his or her feet and then to relax them slowly, or to contract the foot muscles first and then to completely relax them to a point way beyond the starting muscle tension. A third variation is to have the person visualize the feet as loose, molded clay or some similar substance being slowly pulled apart. After spending 30 to 120 seconds with any or all of these descriptions, you then proceed to the lower legs using the same technique. Some people will initially think that they cannot get in touch with the feeling of their feet or legs. You can anticipate this question by telling them first that even though they may think they can't feel their feet, they certainly know exactly what they are wearing on their feet. They know by feeling if they have thin or thick socks on and whether or not they have shoes on. They can tell exactly what kind of surface they're resting on and how far apart their feet are. Similarly, they can feel their legs and know exactly where their socks end. They can feel what type of clothing they have on their legs and they can sense the temperature of the room from the skin of their legs. These cues are invaluable in helping subjects focus in on their muscles (pacing their own muscle tone), so that they can then lead those muscles to greater levels of relaxation.

The exercise is continued with the thighs and then the pelvis and hips. At each point it is necessary to remind the patient to keep up the slow and deep breathing. Continuing upward, have the person focus in on the abdomen, feeling its gentle rising and falling with each breath. At this point you could mention that when watching quiet babies breathe, one can readily see a similar rising and falling of their bellies. Again, time your phrases to the movement of the abdomen. Next comes the back, chest, and shoulders, followed by the arms, forearms, and hands. You can then finish up with the neck and lastly the muscles of the scalp, face, and jaw. Usually each part of the body is taken separately. After practice they can begin to be grouped together as we have just presented.

Certain things in life have to be done precisely the way the manual says. The preceding relaxation exercise is not one of these cases. Some people want to start at the head or with the hands. Some do one side at a time. Those details are not important; in fact, the very act of focused attention (the process) is what leads to the state of relaxation. We suggest you try many combinations— eventually you'll naturally find the one that works best for each individual patient. Some components, however, are indispensable and without them the results will likely be much less powerful. You must remember to continually remind subjects to breathe slowly and deeply (sort of in the way that we keep remining you!). Then, since they'll be breathing in this slow manner, it should be very easy to recognize exactly each inspiration and expiration so as to time the delivery of your phrases with their breaths. You'll also want to slow your talking down as you proceed and begin to talk more softly and deeply. You may wonder whether if you are matching your words to their breaths and if you keep slowing down, they will not eventually turn blue from hyperventilation. The answer, of course, is simply to put fewer words in each breath-matched phrase to create a soothing, relaxing pace.

An experience of one of the authors will illustrate the usefulness of this procedure. A 25-year-old woman came to his office with the following problems. She was alert and oriented but her speech was markedly impaired and her jaw was clenched tight. The author thought that the abnormal speech might have been a chronic condition but the woman and her boyfriend assured him that her speech had been perfectly normal three hours before. She reported that her jaws felt like they were in spasm; indeed, she could only open her mouth about an inch. Her tongue was uncontrollably darting in and out of her mouth in spasms. The perplexed (and frightened) author asked if she were up to date on her tetanus immunizations or if she had incurred any recent cuts on her body. The answer was noncontributory. There was also no history of any drug ingestion. The spasm had come on over a couple of minutes and not suddenly while she was opening her mouth. This fact, plus the physical exam, ruled out dislocation of the temporal-mandibular joint. The only positive finding was the spasm of the tongue and masseter muscles (the muscles of the jaw). Upon further questioning, the woman admitted to an extraordinary amount of tension that was recently placed on her over the last week. She was being asked to work late hours and to be responsible for running her entire office, in which she worked as the secretary. Here was a possible explanation, but the author had never seen this degree of spasm from tension alone. Also, if questioned, almost everyone says they have a lot of tension in some area of their life. (The author did not have one benefit that the reader has, i.e., coming across this case in the middle of a relaxation chapter!) He decided that whatever the problem was, it was doubtful that it would be worsened by a trial of a 15-minute relaxation exercise.

While lying on the table, the patient was instructed in the previously described relaxation process. The author stood at the head of the table with his fingers on the spastic jaw muscles. After some initial uncooperativeness, the patient began to follow the instructions and relax the muscles progressively from her feet upward. The jaw, however, remained in spasm and the darting, spastic tongue seemed to be worse than ever. Probably the most important part of the encounter was that the author did not simply keep saying sentences like, "Your muscles are relaxing beautifully." That definitely would not have paced her experience because she could still feel her spastic jaw and tongue, which certainly were *not* relaxing beautifully. Therefore, very carefully he would say something like, "Your thighs are looking very relaxed and heavy and your jaw is still very tight. You're doing just fine." Most interestingly, each time that he acknowledged the tightness of the jaw, he could feel a momentary, but definite, release of the spasm. He then incorporated this change into his delivery, making her aware that the spasm was no longer in a fixed state but instead a dynamic one.

The author had begun the exercise in a normal tempo. His initial tone probably paced her experience beautifully since there was certainly some fear in it. Gradually, however, by the time they had progressed up to her neck, his voice had deepened and had slowed down to about one third of a normal talking speed. At this point, while the rest of the body looked very relaxed, the tongue was continuing its contortions, although the momentary releases in the jaw were now occurring at a frequency of about every ten seconds. It was at this moment that, while looking down at the woman, the author really experienced her face and suddenly recognized it to be the countenance of a very angry person. He simply said—almost without thinking—"you must be really angry at the way they've been treating you at work." The patient immediately began to sob softly, and simultaneously her jaw and tongue completely released. With the rest of her body feeling relaxed, she had finally felt safe and comfortable enough to let out her true feelings of sadness and frustration. In a normal though tearful voice she related how upset and angry she had been with her boss over the last few days. The spasm did not return at any time in the next few minutes. Afterwards she left the office in a sad but relaxed state.

Reading between the lines it is apparent that another metamorphosis occurred during this interaction. What happens to the moderator of this exercise? First, because a slowing of breathing is suggested to the subject, the moderator will naturally do the same. Voice tempo is then slowed down. When telling the patient to feel her thighs relax, it is very difficult for the moderator to resist that temptation himself. For instance, didn't you just feel that area of your body relax—and again as you read this sentence? By the time the author had progressed to the neck of the patient, he himself was feeling the benefits of the exercise on his body. Probably because of this "grounding" experience, he was better able simply to look down at the woman and see the anger in her face, thereby noticing what was really occurring. This "side effect" of the formal relaxation exercises makes it an even more attractive regimen to keep at our disposal. Remember—patients need to be led into relaxation; no one relaxes on command. One cannot stand over the bed of a child, point his finger, and yell, "Go to sleep!" and expect the child to do so.

At this point, we would like to stress that relaxation techniques are not always the appropriate thing to do with a very anxious patient. For instance, an excited person in the emergency room may benefit from verbal and nonverbal pacing as the specific acute problem is handled. Other times, indirect communication techniques are more helpful. We offer the material in this chapter simply as one other tool for you to have available when interacting with the numerous types of patients you will see.

Teaching Patients Self-Relaxation

Any exercise that our patients use with us, they can learn to use alone. Once the technique is perfected, the time needed will shorten so that within two to five minutes the patient at home can experience a complete loosening up of his or her body. As we have discussed, quite frequently a time may come up in the course of a day when patients start thinking how great it would be to get away and relax. When they can't leave what they are doing, they usually end up resisting the rest of the time they have to be where they are. If instead we encouraged out patients simply to take a five-minute break to loosen all the tight areas of the body, the remaining time spent wherever would be dramatically improved.

The experience of actively relaxing the muscles of the body also enables the patients to take full responsibility for the various aches and pains that they experience throughout the day. Certainly, most people know at some level that when they get a headache it may be coming from a tightness of the scalp and neck muscles. However, at the moment it is first experienced, they are certainly not in touch with this cause and effect. Do we say or think, "Well, I am experiencing pain in the areas of both temples, which must be coming from the fact that I am tightening all the muscles around that area." Of course not! We look up helplessly and say that for some reason we "got a headache," as if a headache were something that just crept into the bloodstream. Or else our teacher gave it to us, or our car, or our lover, spouse or child. This faulty cause-and-effect logic is analogous to watching the sun set in the evening. While we are mesmerized by watching the sun, it might appear that the sun is dropping slowly down behind that part of the earth. Of course, we *know* intellectually that the sun does not ever move and that it's the earth that is rotating. At the moment, however, a slowly moving sun seems very real to us.

What would happen if just once while in the middle of a bad headache your patient were to try a relaxation exercise and be successful in having it disappear? Obviously, he or she would see that the particular surrounding circumstances had remained the same, but that the pain was no longer present. "Out there" could not have been causing the ache over here, or else it would not have left. Seeing the phenomenon from this side now—the side from which there is relaxation and no discomfort—it is much easier for the patient to discover his or her power of control over the pain.

The best way to help patients begin self-relaxation is first to lead them through the process one or several times. Once they experience the gratifying end result, they will find it easier and be much more motivated to start practicing themselves. The following is a delightful example of this.

A middle-aged woman in the office of one of the authors was found on pubic exam to have a moderate-sized vaginal papilloma. One week later she had returned to have it removed. When the author asked her to lie down and put her legs in the stirrups, she said that she was too scared. She said that she wanted to be "put out" or admitted to the hospital for general anesthesia. The author and the nurses reasoned and explained that the only thing she would feel would be the local anesthetic—the actual polyp removal would be painless. However, she continued to refuse. She was obviously too anxious to be reasoned with concerning such a sensitive area. The nurse then suggested using a relaxation technique with the patient. After asking everyone else to leave, the nurse told the patient that since she appeared very tense a relaxation procedure would be used; after becoming more at ease she would then be asked to choose once again. The patient was assured that no one would force her to do anything and that the final decision would be entirely up to her. She then agreed to try the exercise with the nurse. She was first assisted in slowing down her breathing. After this reached a satisfactory level, an awareness of different areas of the body was progressively suggested, all the while continuing to sustain her slowed down breathing. Within three to five minutes she appeared sufficiently relaxed and said that she felt more at ease. The author was called back in and the patient then agreed to get up in the stirrups, providing that she be allowed to come down immediately at any time if it became too scary or painful. The procedure was carried out quickly and uneventfully. But what is also important is that the patient experienced very little observable discomfort during the whole time. What is memorable about the case is that when the patient returned for a routine check up one week later, she exuberantly began relating that in the previous several months she had experienced great difficulty in getting to sleep. Even strong tranquilizers and sleeping pills from her local doctor had proven to be of little value. The night of the polypectomy she experimented with the relaxation exercise to see if it could help her. It was immediately effective and she had continued to use it every night with excellent results.

More than anything else, this last benefit motivates the authors to use these techniques in a regular fashion. In many instances, the relaxation exercises could be replaced by simply injecting a good tranquilizer. However, the great secondary benefits that a patient can reap afterwards would then not be possible. Using the method, the patient has a direct experience that he or she can be comfortable and relaxed regardless of the circumstances. This is a real gift in that there is actually something useful for the patient to take home. This is why whenever we see the possibility of doing such an exercise, we view it as a definite opportunity. Thus our time constraints or other considerations are often overruled in favor of the patient's potential gain. Additionally, patients who are experiencing great fear or pain are the best candidates for this type of exercise. They will put up the least resistance, since they want more than anything to get out of the situation they are in. Thus, besides these patients having the most dramatic and rewarding results, they are often the smoothest responders to the techniques.

Audio Tapes

Taping the exercise regimen for the patient can be very useful. The advantage, of course, is that the health professional need not be present during a practice session at home, but that his or her voice (the anchor to relaxation) is present for the client. An added advantage is that the portable nature of the tape allows it to be used at home, at work, in the hospital room or wherever needed. One example might be a physical therapist who would make tapes for patients and then allow them to play the tapes each day while soaking in a hot tub. A popular practice is to give tapes to patients when they leave the hospital, so that they continue to listen every day. Used in this manner, the tape can be reinforced with actual direct practice sessions when returning as an outpatient.

VISUALIZATION PROCESSES

The Social Service Department of a community hospital in Pittsburgh uses visualization exercises as a relaxation tool for some of its patients. The subject is asked to imagine a scene, such as a quiet lake or a cool forest. As mentioned previously (Chapter 3), when one eidetically visualizes something—seeing it as if from his or her own eyes—it is accompanied by feelings of the same magnitude as when it was originally seen. Leading someone in such a process can be wonderfully relaxing for that person, especially if he or she can visualize eidetically. For those who at first cannot, it is still pleasant and moderately relaxing. With a little practice, eidetic imagery will follow naturally.

Of course, it is a good idea to start this technique in the same fashion as the previous ones; that is, with slow and deep breathing. Another thing to be aware of is to make the story unspecific enough so as to make sure that the person's experience is being paced. If you describe a particular type of yacht and specific types of fish seen through the clear green water, that scene might not match an experience the person has had. The basic principle to remember is never to tell people what they are experiencing. You then leave open the possibility of being wrong and losing your credibility. When talking to patients, be general. For example, if you know the client is visualizing the outside during daytime, you may ask him to look up at the sun. You could then suggest that he notice the time of day by the sun's location. You can safely assume that probably everyone who is visualizing an outside scene during daytime will probably see the sun. You could not safely assume that everyone who is looking outside will see a rainbow, and if you start talking about the specific colors of the rainbow, you will probably lose most patients by being out of pace. So again, the general rule is, be general! At this point, it might be difficult for the subject to visualize eidetically, and a constructed image of such a sight would have to be created. This would not be nearly as effective in eliciting the feelings that are being sought. However, a phrase such as "sitting there watching the water running downstream as the birds chirp away and the sun shines in between the leaves" is much more general, and more likely to be eidetically visualized by someone, since it is a more universal experience.

A variation of this visualization technique is to ask the subject to pick a favorite scene of his or her own, a place in which he or she once felt completely wonderful. A woman in labor who was experiencing a great deal of pain and who was not far enough advanced for pain medication picked a scene in which she was lying with her husband in her backyard looking at the stars on a summer night. From the complete shift in her face and jaw musculature it was easy to see that within about ten seconds she was directly accessing these same feelings that she had experienced in the past. When she came out of the experience about one minute later, the pain had decreased by tenfold.

COMBINING TECHNIQUES

It probably has already occurred to the reader that these techniques can also be combined to produce a very powerful result. For instance, one could start with a traditional muscle relaxing procedure and then proceed to a visualization process. Or else a metaphor could first be presented, followed afterwards with the muscle relaxing exercises. You might note that the metaphors and visualization exercises are very similar. One difference is that, as shown by our own example at the beginning of the chapter, a metaphor can easily be used when the subject might still be tense. A visualization process, since it usually only involves a calm scene, is generally best when the patient has already relaxed a little. However, this is certainly not a steadfast rule, as evidenced in the example of the woman in labor.

An interesting example of the combining of techniques follows. It involves hooking up two relaxation processes by anchoring. It begins by asking a person to recall a particular time when he or she felt really wonderfully relaxed. When this has been accessed fully, it can then be anchored by, for instance, touching an arm. The standard relaxation procedure of body awareness can then be started. The anchor can then be fired at any time, preferably when the observer notices that the patient has become measurably relaxed. The result is usually a shift to a whole new deeper level of relaxation.

The exact procedure was used by one of the authors with a patient in the coronary care unit. He was called there to see a patient who had just gone into paroxysmal atrial tachycardia (P.A.T.).* Immediately, the routine procedures were started: carotid massage, I.V. Tensilon, I.V. digitalis, and I.V. Valium, repeating each of these as indicated. After one hour, the patient was still in the same rhythm. He appeared stable, though somewhat short of breath and very anxious. He related that shortly before the arrhythmia started, the priest had been around to give him last rites. For some strange reason this had upset him, although he was assured when we told him that this was simply what was practiced by the priest on all Catholic ICU patients. His arrhythmia was not as easily convinced and thus continued on.

The patient was asked if he would use a relaxation exercise. He agreed and was told to choose a familiar scene that was very relaxing for him. He picked sitting out on his back porch looking into the woods. This was then anchored. Slow and deep breathing was gradually started, followed by the muscle relaxing exercise. On account of the situation, the procedure was run

---

*A heart arrhythmia in which the heart pumps at twice the normal speed.

through somewhat more quickly than normal. Within a total of two to three minutes the exercise had progressed to his chest; at this point he seemed relaxed enough to fire the anchor. Several seconds after this was done and before the author even had a chance to continue with his shoulders and neck, the author was called to the desk. He instructed the patient to continue to see his relaxing scene and enjoy it and the author left for a minute. When he got to the desk he was told that the patient was now in normal sinus rhythm. The next morning the patient informed the author that he had had a very peaceful night.

CAUSE-AND-EFFECT OR COINCIDENCE?

If you were sitting alone in your room tonight and you suddenly saw a ghost, how many of you would say, "Wow, my first ghost, how exciting!" Most of you would instead begin to wonder what you had been drinking. No doubt some of you would be convinced that you had just become a candidate for the state hospital. In many areas of study, including the health field, there is a tendency to act similarly. We are first taught the way things are and are not. When we later observe things, we see them only through eyes that have filtered these teachings. Thus, when we hear a story such as the last one we often immediately begin to assume that it probably was not the relaxation that made the difference. It must instead have been the I.V. Valium given 40 minutes before, or maybe it just happened to end spontaneously at that moment. . .or perhaps the I.V. Tensilon had just been hanging out in the axillary vein for an hour and finally decided to move on to the heart. What we are suggesting is that you *believe* none of it—that you simply suspend judgment and remember exactly what happened. Perhaps something else will occur that you "knew" wasn't possible. For example, you might see someone's skin rash clear up after one psychotherapy session. If you simply begin to allow things into your awareness in this manner without passing definite judgment as to their validity, you may very well begin to notice a whole new and tremendously exciting stream of events right out there in front of you.

Returning to the subject at hand, we would like to discuss a potential situation you might encounter when doing relaxation exercises. Once in a while a patient may seem not to want to let go of the pleasant scene and feelings—even when you are saying that the session is over and that he should open his eyes. When this happens, it is important to allow the patient the extra time needed and let him know that he can open his eyes whenever he finishes, whether it be in two minutes or five minutes or even ten minutes. (This is a perfect time for the old illusion of choice method.) Usually even this is not necessary, because if you are successfully pacing him with your tonal output, the patient will know when to stop. When describing a blue sky, the clear water, and the gentle breeze, ideally your voice will be slow and soothing. As you draw the exercise to a close, your voice should begin to return to its normal tonality. This will serve as a nonverbal lead in redirecting the patient to his normal state of awareness. You also can and should remind the patient that the relaxation is a state that he created himself and that he can recreate it at any time. The ability to relax is not limited to your office space and time. The important thing to realize is that if the patient stays in his relaxed state, it is because he is choosing to because of the good feelings. Some people have reported being angry when told to come out of their scene, saying, for instance, "It was *my* scene. I didn't want you telling me when I had to leave!" The idea we are attempting to convey is simply not to get excited in the situation in which this may occur—the patient is not going to get stuck there forever. Simply recognize that the person is demanding more time and go along with it. You can sometimes even utilize such a happening and ask the patient to find a spot in the scene to take a short nap for five or ten minutes, thereafter awakening refreshed and alert.

In concluding the chapter, we would like to return to the example of the patient with the polyp. The manner in which we view the whole encounter is that by assisting her in relaxing we were simply helping her to have an alternative. Before the exercise, all she could do was experience her fear and tension. She was literally immobilized and could not even consider moving up into the stirrups. She could only experience all of her previous pictures of doctors, doctors' offices, scalpels, blood, and so on. By offering her an alternative—relaxation—we opened up new choices for her. She was then able to hear us more clearly when we told her there would be hardly any pain involved. She could then choose: Did she want to enter the hospital and leave her family for a couple of days, risk general anesthesia, pay more money — or instead at least first try the exercise in the office. She *herself* chose first to try the exercise and then to have the surgery in the office. She benefited, in that the experience was virtually atraumatic and in turn assisted her in terminating her four-month history of insomnia. For those who want to call it manipulation, that's okay. We realize that these techniques probably could be used for self-interest motives. Hopefully, the people who read this book and use the techniques will be interested in goals that are consistent with the well-being of the patients whom they serve. For instance, the drugs we give patients certainly invade and manipulate different biochemical systems in their bodies. Many of them even cause a fair number of adverse side effects. We use them anyway, since the potential benefit they offer overrides the relative risk. When an osteopath or chiropractor cracks someone's back, that's also manipulation (they even call it that!). A physical therapist massaging someone's neck to loosen the taut musculature there is performing a smiliar process.

As usual, reading about relaxation—or skiing or sex—just doesn't make it in the experiential universe. Do a few of these techniques by yourself and with your friends or classmates. Once you have experienced the remarkable clarity and well-being that can be achieved in this state, you will enthusiastically want to share it with your patients.

When using the various relaxation techniques, you may at first notice a tendency of the patient to feel drowsy or even to fall asleep during the exercise. Some people enjoy this—the level of sleep is actually a very light, often dream-associated experience. Others would rather stay awake. With practice, most people can learn to remain conscious. This can be facilitated by the use of certain supportive techniques such as sitting in a chair that has a straight back and no head support. Some people may always experience falling asleep. For them, simply realize that they are choosing to utilize this unconscious level in order to attain the greatest degree of relaxation that is available to them.

We sincerely hope that no one thinks we have presumed to have covered the market on relaxation. For some, it can come as easily as stooping down to pet a cat or smiling at a baby. For others, it simply means talking with a friend. The job of the health professional is to help patients find their best way to relax and to encourage them to use it.

EXERCISES

1. Discuss areas of your clinical practice, as well as your personal life, in which relaxation exercises could be useful.
2. Practice relaxation exercises with your partners. Experiment with each of the techniques we have presented.

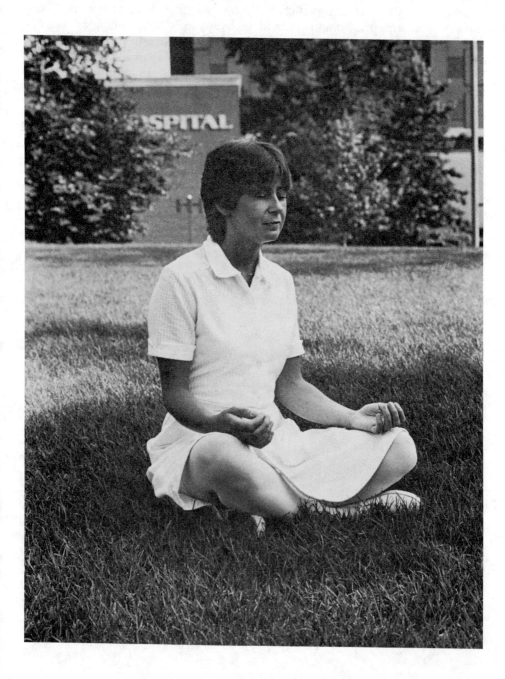

And Remember 10

And a woman spoke, saying, "Tell us of Pain."
And he said . . . "Much of your pain is self-chosen. It is the bitter potion by which
the physician within you heals your sick self.
"Therefore trust the physician and drink his remedy in silence and tranquility. . . ."

Kahlil Gibran, *The Prophet*

REFERENCES AND SELECTED BIBLIOGRAPHY

Abbott, E.: *Flatland: A Romance in Many Dimensions,* 6th edition. New York: Dover, 1952.

Bandler, R., and Grinder, J.: *The Structure of Magic,* Vols. I and II. Palo Alto, Ca.: Science and Behavior Books, 1975.

Bandler, R., and Grinder, J.: *Patterns of the Hypnotic Techniques of Milton H. Erickson, M.D.* Cupertino, Ca.: Meta Publications, 1975.

Bandler, R., and Grinder, J.: *Frogs Into Princes.* Moab, Utah: Real People Press, 1979.

Bandler, R., Grinder, J., and Satir, V.: *Changing with Families.* Palo Alto, Ca.: Science and Behavior Books, 1976.

Bateson, G.: *Mind and Nature: A Necessary Unit.* New York: E. P. Dutton, 1979.

Bateson, G., Jackson, D., Haley, J., and Weakland, J. H.: Toward a theory of schizophrenia. *Behavioral Sciences,* 1:251–264, 1956.

Bettelheim, B.: *The Uses of Enchantment.* New York: Random House, 1975.

Blondis, M. N., and Jackson, B. E.: *Nonverbal Communication with Patients.* New York: John Wiley and Sons, 1977.

Cameron-Brandler, L.: *They Lived Happily Ever After.* Cupertino, Ca.: Meta Publications, 1978.

Erickson, M. H., and Rossi, E.: *Hypnotherapy Casebook.* New York: Irvington, 1979.

Erickson, M. H., Rossi, E., and Rossi, S.: *Hypnotic Realities.* New York: Irvington, 1976.

Gibran, K.: *The Prophet.* New York: Alfred Knopf Inc., 1923.

Gordon, D.: *Therapeutic Metaphors.:* Cupertino, Ca.: Meta Publications, 1978.

Haley, J., ed.: *Advanced Techniques of Hypnosis and Therapy: Selected Papers of Milton H. Erickson, M.D.* New York: Grune & Stratton, 1967.

Haley, J.: *Uncommon Therapy, The Psychiatric Techniques of Milton H. Erickson, M.D.* New York: Norton, 1973.

Lankton, S. R.: *Practical Magic: The Clinical Applications of Neuro-Linguistic Programming.* Cupertino, Ca.: Meta Publications, 1979.

Riley, V.: Mouse mammary tumors: alleviation of incidence as apparent function of stress." *Science,* 189:465–467, 1975.

Roberts, S. L.: *Behavioral Concepts and the Critically Ill Patient.* Englewood Cliffs, N.J.: Prentice Hall, 1976.

Rosenthal, R.: The use of film in measuring sensitivity to nonverbal communication: the PONS test. Paper presented at the 81st annual convention, American Psychological Association, Montreal, August 1973.

Solomon, G. F., and Amkraut, A. A.: Emotions, stress, and immunity. *Frontiers of Radiation Therapy and Oncology,* 7:84–96, 1972.

Watzlawick, P.: *How Real Is Real?* New York: Random House, 1976.

Watzlawick, P.: *The Language of Change.* New York: Norton, 1978.

Index